THERAPEUTIC CAREGIVING:

*A Practical Guide for
Caregivers of Persons with
Alzheimer's and Other
Dementia-Causing Diseases*

THERAPEUTIC CAREGIVING:

A Practical Guide for Caregivers of Persons with Alzheimer's and Other Dementia-Causing Diseases

Barbara J. Bridges, R.N.,
M.S.N., M.S.H.C.M., M.B.A.

BJB Publishing
Mill Creek, Washington

Illustrations by: Jaime Temairik

Publisher's Cataloging in Publication

Bridges, Barbara J.
  Therapeutic caregiving: a practical guide for caregivers of persons with
  Alzheimer's and other dementia-causing diseases / Barbara J. Bridges—
  2nd rev. ed.
  p. cm.
  ISBN 0-9645178-0-9

  1. Dementia—Patients—Care—Handbooks, manuals, etc. 2. Alzheimer's
  disease—Patients—Care—Handbooks, manuals, etc. 3. Parkinsonism—
  Patients—Care—Handbooks, manuals, etc. 4. Cerebrovascular disease—
  Patients—Care—Handbooks, manuals, etc. 5. Nursing—Care—Hand-
  books, manuals, etc. 6. Home care—home care nursing, etc.
  I. Title.

  RC521.B75 1995   618.8'3
                                                    QBI95-10058

Copyright: © 1995, 1996, 1998   Barbara J. Bridges
First Printing: 1995   **BJB PUBLISHING**
Second Printing: 1996, revised   16212 Bothell Way S.E., Suite F171
Third Printing: 1998   Mill Creek, Washington 98012-1219
                                       (800) 799-3414

Printed and bound in the United States of America
Third Printing: 1998
Library of Congress Catalog Card Number: 95-94060
ISBN 0-9645178-0-9

DEDICATION

This book is dedicated to the loving memory of:

- ➤ my father, Walter Bridges;

- ➤ my dear and caring mother, Elsie Nelsen Bridges;

- ➤ and my best friend and adult lifelong companion,
  Dr. Bruce F. Baisch,

all of whom developed some form of dementing illness in their aging years. By working closely with each of them, I have been able to develop and experiment with techniques and interventions that they and I found to be most useful.

Mother was especially patient with me—patient with my numerous inquiries as to what worked and what didn't work, and what made her feel better or what made her feel worse. Mother experienced both extremely confused periods as well as periods when she was more lucid and, fortunately, was able to express what she was feeling during the previous confused period. From our shared experiences we each gained a great deal, both in knowledge of approaches that succeeded and failed, and in emotional closeness.

TABLE OF CONTENTS

PREFACE

This book is intended to be a down-to-earth practical guide for caregivers of persons with dementing illness. The term *"caregivers"* is utilized in referring to any relative, friend, neighbor, or employed person who is providing assistance to a person having difficulty functioning due to cognitive impairment—the impaired ability to think and make appropriate judgments. Caregivers are those who are providing on-site support as well as those who occasionally look in on or telephone someone with dementing illness—anyone who interacts with the person.

This book is experience based, rather than research based, although nursing concepts contained herein are grounded in research. I am a registered nurse who, for over 14 years, not only provided care for both of my parents and my best friend who had dementia, but also has counseled friends and relatives finding themselves thrust into the caregiving situation. Clients in my private practice and Alzheimer's Association support group members have provided me with rich experiences, as well. It is my hope that information in this book is provided in such a way that it can be easily understood and utilized not only by untrained caregivers, such as family members, but also by trained caregivers delivering services in the home, retirement homes, assisted living units, adult family homes, and in other long term care environments.

Many books have been written that address the diseases that cause dementia and the nature and course of dementia, itself.

Others address the need for respite and caring for the care-givers. Several books which will supplement and complement this book are found in the complementary resource section, Appendix A, at the back of the book.

This book, however, is quite different. It is written with primary consideration for the person with dementia. I have tried consistently, in working closely with parents, relatives, friends, and clients with dementia to place myself in the shoes of the person with the problem. The techniques I have learned and the information I am presenting in this book emanate directly from the information I have gleaned from persons with dementing illness. I believe it is only through my prolonged, intense, and intimate relationships with these persons that I have been able to experience and learn the techniques presented herein.

I fully recognize that I, as an educated nursing professional, leave myself open to criticism from colleagues in publishing information that is not research based. However, I believe the very nature of the dementia process and what it does to one's cognitive capacity makes research difficult, at best. It has been my observation that persons with dementing illness function much better in familiar environments, without the presence of strangers or stressful situations. Visiting a physician, psychologist, nurse, social worker, or other health care professional for evaluation and/or treatment may be stressful enough to cause the person with dementing illness, who already has diminished-cognitive capacity, to test at a lower functional level.

The above observations on testing are not meant to discourage seeking appropriate early and on-going evaluation and treatment for the person with signs of cognitive impairment. Testing, however, may result in an inaccurate assessment of the capabilities of the person with dementia—especially in the areas of function that count most for the caregiver and the person with dementing illness—that is the person's ability to live and function in a familiar environment in this complicated world with a reasonable quality of life.

I believe the only place to accurately evaluate the person's ability to perform activities necessary to remain active and independent is in his/her familiar environment, whether it be at home, with family, or in another type of care unit. Evaluating the ability of the person with dementia to carry out normal activities of daily living and making plans to assist the person to continue to live an active and rewarding life are primary responsibilities of caregivers and the real mission of caregiving.

It is my wish, then, that this book will provide dedicated caregivers with information which will assist them in their very difficult roles of providing day-in and day-out support and therapeutic caring to person's with dementia, thereby enhancing this aging person's quality of life. If nothing more, I hope that by reading this book, caregivers may be stimulated to creatively design programs that will work effectively both for them and for the recipients of their skilled and nurturing services. I further hope that, by enhancing the skill level of caregivers, they will find some sense of satisfaction and reward in providing seemingly thankless services for clients, friends, or loved ones.

Special Note to Readers:

I intentionally have not included an index in this book. The material is organized in such a way that if portions or chapters are skipped, many sequentially provided concepts will be missed. I suggest you read the book completely before seeking information on specific topics, then utilize the detailed Table of Contents.

ACKNOWLEDGMENTS

My profound thanks to Burton V. Reifler, M.D., M.P.H., Professor and Chairman, Department of Psychiatry and Behavioral Medicine, Bowman Gray School of Medicine, Wake Forest University, and to Eric B. Larson, M.D., Medical Director, University of Washington Medical Center, and principle investigator for the Alzheimer's Disease Research Center, University of Washington. Their review of contents from a medical research perspective was invaluable.

My thanks, also, to Howard Gruetzner, M.Ed., Director of Elder Services, Heart of Texas Region Mental Health and Mental Retardation, for his critical review of the original manuscript. Howard's book, *Alzheimer's: A Caregiver's Guide and Sourcebook,* is referenced in Appendix A in the back of this book.

I am deeply indebted to my nursing colleagues, Carol Mills, R.N., M.A., Sandra Pflaum, R.N., M.S.N., and Karen Strand, M.A., R.N., for their professional input and review.

Thanks also to Jaime Temairik, a Mukilteo, Washington, high school art student, for her many hours of work on illustrations for the exercise segments.

I also wish to thank Mary Ann Wilson, R.N., President, *Sit and Be Fit*™, *Inc.*, Spokane, Washington, for her conscientious review of the exercise content of this book. Mary Ann's highly acclaimed senior fitness program can be viewed on PBS television stations nationwide.

My sincerest thanks to many of my friends and relatives who so generously gave of their time and skills to read and critique chapters of this book as they were written.

Finally, a special thank you to all of the members of the Alzheimer's Association Support Group in Edmonds, Washington. You were invaluable not only in critiquing my written manuscript, but also in allowing me to teach many of the techniques incorporated within. Your willingness to share your experiences has enriched my life and provided added dimension to this book.

1

DEMENTIA: AN OVERVIEW

Dementia Defined

Simply put, *"dementia"* means the loss of or impairment of mental functioning. Symptoms include memory loss, confusion, disorientation, intellectual impairment, and general loss of reasoning ability. Dementia is not a disease, but rather a condition which may be brought on by a myriad of diseases. Some diseases that cause symptoms of dementia are treatable. However, this book is written for caregivers of those with dementing illness which is irreversible.

The term *"cognitive impairment"* is utilized throughout this book. Cognitive impairment refers to a person's diminished capacity to think, reason, and make appropriate decisions. More specifically, a person with cognitive impairment is unable to utilize appropriate judgment and thought processes.

Among diseases which result in dementia, or dementia-like symptoms, are Alzheimer's disease, and multi-infarct disease, sometimes referred to as vascular disease of the brain. Multi-infarct disease is a series of mini-strokes or clots in blood vessels in the brain. Approximately 50% of all persons with irreversible dementia have Alzheimer's disease. Another 20-25% have multi-infarct disease. Additionally, approximately 20% of persons with dementia have the combination of Alzheimer's disease and multi-infarct disease. The remaining 5-10% of persons with dementing illness are suffering from numerous other neurological diseases, including Parkinson's disease and Picks disease. Recent statistics indicate nearly half of Americans over the age of 85 have dementing illness. It is estimated that somewhere between 80 and 90 percent of these people are cared for in their homes or in homes of relatives by loving spouses, other family members, or employed caregivers.

Normal Course of Dementia

Each person with dementing illness displays a somewhat individualized set of symptoms. Additionally, the speed with which the degree of dementia increases varies with each individual. Generally, persons with Alzheimer's disease have a very slow onset of symptoms, progressing gradually over an extended period of time. Persons with multi-infarct disease generally have a more sudden onset of the condition, which may either stabilize at one level, or progress to other levels in step-wise fashion with each disturbance of blood vessels in the brain. Frequently, diseases causing dementia are all present. Other chronic diseases common to the aging adult, such as heart disease, respiratory disease, hypertension, and vascular disease may be present, as well. Therefore, providing care for persons with dementing illness is a complex and difficult undertaking.

Dementia usually starts with difficulty with functions of the mind, but nearly always ends in gradual loss of ability to function physically, including performance of normal activities of daily living, such as eating, bathing, dressing, etc. The loss of mental and physical functioning may occur gradually over 10 to 15 years or more, or more rapidly, depending on the underlying cause of the problem and the age at onset of the dementia process. Early onset dementing illness, that is, illness which is diagnosed before age 65 tends to progress a little more rapidly than does that which becomes evident after age 65.

This **terrifying** loss of ability to function is usually recognized, but not always acknowledged, by the person with dementia. Frequently, the person finds ways to cover for losses of mental functioning. Additionally, family members or friends may step in and take over to cover the problem. Furthermore, family members or friends may deny the problem exists, leaving the person with dementing illness without appropriate assistance and support, and a tremendous amount of fear.

Persons with dementing illness may begin to withdraw socially and may have a clinical depression contributing to the symptoms, as well. The sense of loss of mental and physical capacity to think for and/or care for oneself becomes all consuming. Frequently, persons with dementia are in such a state of denial or deep fear that they will say everything is fine. Others may be crying for assistance by making such comments as: "I can't remember anything anymore;" or "No one wants to talk with me;" or "I'm getting so forgetful;" or "What will others think of me?" Some may joke about their memory loss as an off-beat way of asking for help.

It is extremely important for family members, friends, or health care professionals who hear comments such as those described above, or observe signs and symptoms of memory loss to take appropriate action to prevent the person with possible dementing illness from becoming frightened. Action would include honest discussion with the loved one or patient, and planning for a full geriatric assessment to determine if a problem exists, and if so, if it is treatable. How frightening it would be to be constantly asking for help and be ignored by loved ones or health care professionals.

Health care professionals have developed some tools or scales for measuring the degree of cognitive impairment in a person with dementia. One popular scale in use today is the seven stage "Global Deterioration Scale" developed by Dr. Barry Reisburg, Clinical Director of the Aging and Dementia Research Center at New York University. However, an individual with dementia may display behaviors from several of the stages at varying times during the disease process, making classification relatively meaningless from the caregiver's perspective. Those of us who are or have been caregivers for persons with dementia know that cognitive abilities change throughout the day, hour, week, or month. There can be periods of clarity in thinking and periods of confusion. Caregivers do need to understand the general nature of the decline which will result from dementia-causing diseases. More important, however, is the need for concrete information on how to manage situations and behaviors that arise as a result of the disease process, regardless of the person's place on a cognitive impairment scale. In short, except for gaining an understanding of what to expect with your loved one with dementia, classification schemes are relatively meaningless from the caregiver's perspective.

Those of you who are just beginning to face the problem of being a caregiver for someone with dementia may read this book and say, "I don't see these behaviors in my loved one." It is entirely

possible that some of the behaviors described in this book, in
other publications, or in classification scales, may never occur.
However, the most important aspect a caregiver can bring to
this situation of caregiving is the knowledge of what might happen, along with the stamina and fortitude to address the early
symptoms of problems head-on and in a forthright manner. To
the extent that early signs of problems are addressed as described in this book, the caregiver has an opportunity to delay
and/or even prevent the onset of some of the disastrous consequences of dementia causing diseases. Problem prevention is a
major function of therapeutic caregivers.

The Importance of a Thorough Evaluation

Some persons with treatable physical illnesses may display
dementia-like symptoms. Therefore, it is important for persons
with these symptoms to be evaluated by a competent geriatric
assessment team consisting minimally of a geriatric internist,
geriatric psychiatrist, geriatric social worker, geriatric nutrition-
ist, geriatric clinical pharmacologist, and geriatric nurse to rule
out treatable medical conditions and/or confirm the presence of a
specific disease causing the dementia condition. Usually, geriatric assessment teams are housed at major metropolitan teaching
medical centers.

Don't expect your loved one with symptoms of dementing illness
to request to be evaluated. The very nature of the dementing
process prevents one from thinking logically. Additionally, denial and fear are prevalent feelings of the person who realizes
he/she is losing the ability to think. Usually, loving family members have to insist on an evaluation. The nature and degree of
discussion with your loved one depends on the willingness of the
person to agree and/or cooperate. With a cooperative loved one,

full discussion is best and develops trust. If your loved one will become agitated and resist evaluation, making the appointment without in-depth discussion and simply taking the person may be the best approach.

The caregiver becomes the major advocate and spokesperson for the person with dementia during this evaluation process. Documentation of physical and mental problems observed by the caregiver may be the only accurate information a physician or other health professional can utilize in evaluating and treating the person with dementing illness. The caregiver must apprise the health care professional of the severity of the person's loss of mental functioning and correct any misinformation given directly to the health care professional by the person with dementia.

Treatment for Dementia

There currently is no effective cure for either the diseases that cause irreversible dementia or the dementia condition itself. Some medications, nevertheless, may improve either mental or physical functioning. However, other chronic diseases and conditions which affect the over-all physical and mental well-being of the individual may be treatable. Therefore, it is extremely important to be on the alert for any symptoms of physical illness or depression which are readily treatable, and which can make life more comfortable for the person with dementing illness. Additionally, improving visual or auditory functions by obtaining or maintaining glasses or hearing aids, may improve cognitive social functioning.

Is Dementia the Same as Senility?

The term *"senility"* has been utilized for years by those in the medical community and the lay public to define an array of conditions attributed to old age. Senility is a general term which has no medical meaning or definition, and the unfortunate consequence of its use has been the ongoing belief that senility is a normal process of aging and that problems that generate symptoms of senility are untreatable. Since we now know that many treatable diseases and illnesses generate symptoms lumped into this previously utilized "senility" category, the use of this term should be avoided.

There is a growing body of knowledge which defines appropriate methods for working with persons with dementing illness—methods which will foster and encourage independence of these persons in both physical and mental functioning. It is to this important role of the caregiver, whether a professional or family member, that the information incorporated herein is directed.

2

THE THERAPEUTIC ROLE OF THE CAREGIVER

Managing Feelings and Role Change Problems

This segment is directed toward the family member caregiver of a person with dementia. What is your role in this very difficult situation in which you find yourself? At first glance, the answer seems obvious. You simply will see that your loved one gets kind and loving care.

Many other books, some of which are referenced at the back of this book, address caregiver feelings and the need for support and respite. Therefore, I will not address these problems at length. However, until you are a caregiver in this new and strange role, it is very difficult to conceive the tremendous numbers of role problems and major lifestyle changes you will face.

What if you are used to depending on your spouse to perform financial activities? What if you always depended upon your mother or father to be there for you? What if your grandmother always knew what to do? What will you feel the first time you have to actually assist your loved one with toileting? What will you feel the first time your loved one doesn't seem to know your name, or what your relationship is?

The objective response to all of the above questions is that your loved one can no longer perform in these roles. I can tell you from personal experience, however, that it is extremely hard to believe and accept what can happen when dementing illness starts decreasing the cognitive capabilities of your loved one's mind. You are literally observing a slow and ongoing death of your loved one. We, as human beings living in a highly techno-logical society, are not generally equipped to manage any situa-tion for which there is no cure or quick fix.

If you are/become intimately involved in daily caregiving, you will not believe the horrendous nightmare you and your loved one will be facing as the dementing illness progresses. Minimal-ly, you will experience feelings of anger, frustration, fright, insecurity, pity, sadness, and depression. It is extremely easy for family member caregivers to become totally bogged down with feelings—feelings about themselves and feelings about their loved ones. I certainly do not desire to discount these feelings—they are real! Deal with them in support groups, through discussions with friends and family, or seek profession-al or spiritual counselling.

Where to Get Support

I strongly recommend becoming involved in a support group of other caregivers of persons with dementing illness. These groups may be available through churches, nursing homes, retirement homes or other community services. However, the groups I recommend most are those sponsored by the Alzheimer's Association. The local chapter phone number is usually listed in the white pages of your telephone directory. If not, contact the national organization. The phone number is in Appendix A, at the end of this book.

These support groups provide not only a source of knowledge about dementia causing illnesses, but also, and more importantly, an opportunity to share in the experiences and camaraderie of others who are facing the devastation of living with and working with a loved one deteriorating with dementing illness.

One of the reasons I recommend support groups of others experiencing similar caregiving situations is that, as a support group facilitator, I hear over and over again that family members or friends who have not experienced this painful process of caregiving simply "do not understand." Family members tend to avoid communication with both the person with dementing illness and that person's caregiver. If communication occurs, non-caregivers say things like, "Oh, he looks so good," or "She walks so well." Persons with dementing illness can look great and physically do fairly well until very late in the disease process, but comments related to physical abilities avoid the real issue—the loss of cognitive capacity—the problem necessitating caregiving in the first place. Given a choice of losing our ability to walk versus losing our ability to think and reason, I suspect most of us would choose the former.

Other comments you may hear from friends, family members, or even other caregivers relate to the state of being of the person with dementia. "He doesn't know you," or "She doesn't know the difference," are frequently heard comments. These statements simply assume the person with dementing illness has no mind at all, and, therefore, cannot think or have feelings. These comments, in essence, imply that the caregiver should ignore his/her loved one, since he/she doesn't know the difference anyway. Nothing could be farther from the truth. Persons with dementing illness are even more sensitive than many of us who are not cognitively impaired. They are thinking, feeling human beings with needs and desires just like the rest of us. Unfortunately, they can't consistently communicate their needs to those of us functioning in the "fast track" world in which we live.

My rationale for dwelling on these seemingly negative issues is that the myriad of feelings discussed in preceding paragraphs are exacerbated by the insensitive comments of many people around us. Caregivers frequently find themselves not only facing an emotionally and physically draining situation, but also, comments and behaviors from others who are unintentionally less than supportive.

One would like to think that providing non-caregivers with knowledge about the disease process and caregiver problems would change attitudes and behaviors. However, it has been my personal experience, and that of many other caregivers, that educating family members and friends not directly involved on a day-to-day basis may have little effect. Perhaps their attitudes and comments, which are so aggravating for emotionally and physically stressed caregivers, are mechanisms of denial, anger, and/or anxiety.

What caregivers need are support and respite. Unfortunately, what caregivers frequently receive are insensitivity and avoidance by those who could be emotionally supportive and offer respite or relief for the caregiver. Therefore, it is extremely important to find a sensitive and understanding person or persons, whether they be family, friends, clergy, professional counselors, or support group members, to provide emotional and spiritual support. This information is not meant to criticize or diminish the loving and kind support provided by many relatives and friends of caregivers. Rather it serves to warn caregivers that family members and friends may not always be supportive. I don't know how I would have survived the last several years without the loving support of my brother and a few close friends and family members, many of whom have faced similar caregiving situations.

Summarizing, caregivers need to work through their feelings in whatever way is appropriate for them so they can manage the ever increasing challenges ahead.

The Therapeutic Role

What I am suggesting in this book is that caregivers begin looking at themselves in a new light—one of providing therapeutic care for their loved ones. I submit that getting bogged down with feelings accomplishes nothing. Rather, caregivers need to get themselves into a problem solving mode. This mode is not feeling driven, it is solution driven.

Prevention of problems is the primary role of the therapeutic caregiver. Obtaining knowledge and skills in caregiving for persons with dementia is crucial to performing problem prevention activities. Some of these essential caregiver skills are more practical than they are theoretical in nature. Others are based on nursing research and practice, but easily learned by family member caregivers.

I realize there has been very little assistance heretofore regarding what caregivers can do for a loved one with dementia. The contents of this book will give you some concrete tools to aid you in performing your new role—the role of therapeutic caregiver for the person with dementing illness.

3

MISSION, PHILOSOPHY, AND GOALS OF CAREGIVING

Mission of Caregiving

The major mission of caregiving is to promote independence, by maintaining the person with dementia in his/her most functional state—physically, intellectually, emotionally, and spiritually.

Philosophy

The major philosophical approach and the justification for all caregiver decisions must be based on a reverence for life, and the belief that human beings have the innate right to function to their highest level of mental and physical capacity. The fact that the person with dementing illness needs assistance from a caregiver does not diminish that right. This philosophy will engender in the person a continuing sense of achievement and well-being, in spite of his/her diminishing intellectual, emotional, and physical capacities. .

Our society has a difficult time dealing with problems that affect the mind. The highest level of physical and mental independence will occur, however, only by active evaluation and problem solving which include the person with the disease condition. Problem prevention and/or resolution must be confronted openly, honestly, and objectively. If a loved one, client, or patient had a physical problem, (e.g., a broken leg), we would have no difficulty in discussing the problem with the injured person and designing solutions to make the person more functional, independent, and comfortable.

This same matter-of-fact approach works extremely well with persons with dementing illness. It has been my experience that the person with the disease is quite aware of his/her problems, even before they are observed by a loved one, caregiver or health care professional. Usually, directness and honesty are met with a tremendous amount of relief. To the extent that the person with dementia can develop a sense of trust of the caregiver or professional, the inevitable and increasing problems that most assuredly will occur as a result of the disease process can be dealt with much more readily and pleasantly.

Goals

It is important for the caregiver not only to think philosophically about his/her beliefs about caring for the person with dementia, but also to develop specific goals which will serve to enhance the life of the person who is the recipient of care. I have identified a few general goals for the caregiver to consider, along with supporting rationale. Detailed explanations are woven throughout the text of this book.

- To maintain a lifestyle as close as possible to the lifestyle of the person pre-dementia.

  One of the most prevalent problems for the person with dementing illness is increasing difficulty in adapting to change. Therefore, the caregiver must do everything realistically feasible to maintain a lifestyle as close as possible to that which the person lived pre-dementia. The person with dementia will remain functional longer when assisted by the caregiver to perform activities, schedules, and routines that were customary prior to contracting the dementia-causing disease. Additional benefits will ensue from keeping the person in a familiar environment such as his/her own home or that of a loved one.

  Environment is the key variable here. Due to decreased ability to adapt to changes or different environments, the person with dementia will remain functional longer if kept in a familiar environment with appropriate assistance provided by a caregiver.

- To promote independent physical functioning to the highest level possible.

  It goes without saying that we all want to be active physically and able to do as much for ourselves as is possible. Due to the physically degenerative nature of dementia-causing diseases, this goal is extremely important to the person with dementia. Additionally, performing normal physical activities of living aids in promoting a sense of self-worth, subsequently addressed.

◆ To promote independent mental functioning to the highest
   level possible.

   The most worrisome and frightening problem for the person
   with dementia is that of coping with the reality that his/her
   mind is slipping away. I have talked with numerous people
   with dementia who have just come into a more lucid moment
   after having had a period of confusion. When asked if they
   were feeling "mad," "sad," "glad," or "afraid," invariably the
   response was "afraid." I believe caregivers can consciously
   assist the thinking processes and stimulate the minds of
   those with dementia. Techniques will be discussed throughout the remainder of this book.

◆ To promote a feeling of self-worth.

   Our society rewards those with "good" minds. It is hard to
   feel good about yourself when you know you are losing your
   ability to think. However, the caregiver can greatly influence
   how the person with dementia perceives his/her value. By
   assisting the person in performing both productive and social
   activities, rewarding appropriate behavioral responses, and
   encouraging others to do likewise, the caregiver can enhance
   the self-worth of the person with dementing illness.

◆ To provide a safe environment.

   Knowing that the person with dementia loses thinking and
   judging abilities, it becomes the caregiver's responsibility to
   be certain the environment in which the recipient functions
   is safe. Safety includes making decisions and taking actions
   which prevent unsafe situations for the person with dementia and for others, including caregivers.

◆   To provide for privacy.

Some of us are extremely social in nature. Others of us need a lot of "alone" time to regroup and regain our sense of self. All of us need some time to regroup. The very nature of the decline as a result of dementia-causing diseases necessitates more and more close contact and assistance by others. Persons with dementia need private time away from the constant bombardment of direction and stimulation from caregivers or social situations. Caregivers need to provide for some private time for the person with dementia.

◆   To provide for social contact with friends and relatives.

One of the dynamics of human nature is that we communicate with and socialize with people who are responsive to us. Given the nature of decline in social abilities of persons with dementia, providing for essential contact and communication with family members and friends becomes increasingly difficult. As the person with dementia becomes less communicative, others respond by distancing themselves. The caregiver can be of great assistance in enhancing socialization skills, so the person will not feel rejected and abandoned.

◆   To provide a nurturing and caring environment.

The increased sensitivity of the person with dementia to moods and feelings of others has been observed by many family caregivers. This more sensitive person will quickly detect a hostile or uncaring atmosphere. The caregiver must provide both a caring as well as a nurturing environment. The term *"nurturing"* is utilized here in the physical, mental, and spiritual sense.

These goals, then, serve to emphasize and enhance the over-all mission of caregiving. Establishing specific plans to meet these general goals will do much to foster the functioning and well-being of the person with dementia.

4

THE NEED FOR A FUNCTIONAL EVALUATION

The evaluation to which I am referring in this section is a functional evaluation of the capabilities of the person with dementia to carry out routines and activities of daily living. This evaluation would follow the in-depth medical evaluation by a team of geriatric specialists. This evaluation would take place only after there has been a previous determination that the person has an irreversible dementia-causing disease such as Alzheimer's disease, multi-infarct disease, or Parkinson's disease.

A carefully considered philosophy of care and well planned goals cannot be implemented without this functional evaluation. Not only is there a need for initial evaluation as a basis for formulating the plan of care, but also, there is a need for ongoing evaluation to determine progress made or extent of disease related deterioration in the performance of activities of daily living. In other words, this evaluation starts the goal planning process.

It is important that the evaluation be performed and the plan of care established by someone with geriatric assessment skills. A geriatric nursing specialist is ideal for this type of evaluation. The best plan of care will be determined through discussion with the geriatric practitioner making the assessment, the person with dementia, and all family, friends, and caregivers who have had an opportunity to observe the person with dementia. Obtaining appropriate input from other health professionals such as the person's physician, a psychiatrist, psychologist, social worker, physical therapist, occupational therapist, or speech therapist will be beneficial, as well.

The evaluation and subsequent plan of care must include minimally:

◆ A total physical and mental capability assessment.

◆ A determination of which activities of daily living (personal care activities) can be done independently, and which activities require cueing (either written or verbal).

   Note: The concept of cueing will be discussed in depth in subsequent chapters.

◆ A determination of changes in procedures, and/or environment that are essential for safety.

◆ A determination of what mentally stimulating activities are appropriate.

◆ A determination of appropriate physical exercise to maintain posture, balance, strength, and endurance.

- A determination of what activities of daily living or recreational activities the person can be trained or retrained to perform, either with some cueing or independently.

- Specific written cue sequences for all activities requiring assistance of the caregiver, both for verbal cues and for written cues.

- A written daily schedule of activities.

- A written schedule of weekly, or monthly activities which need to be performed.

- Provision for periodic review and revision of the plan of care to meet the changing needs of the person with dementing illness.

The person responsible for health care provided to the person with dementia must continually evaluate activities of the caregivers to be certain there is consistency and adherence to the plan of care. Additionally, the person with dementia must be evaluated on a ongoing basis to determine level of improvement or of deterioration, each of which would necessitate changing the plan of care.

5

COMMUNICATING WITH THE PERSON WITH DEMENTIA

A major skill caregivers of persons with dementing illness must learn is that of how to adapt communication so that persons with a damaged brain can participate in the communication process. Failure to learn this skill, or more appropriately, this series of skills, will result in much frustration in both the person with dementing illness and the caregiver.

"Imagine forgetting the beginning of this sentence by the time you reach the end." This sentence, credited to the Alzheimer's Association of Western and Central Washington Chapter of the national Alzheimer's Disease and Related Disorders Association, Inc., provides insight into cognitive functioning problems of the person with dementing illness. This sentence is particularly relevant to determining potential problems in communicating with persons with cognitive impairment. Caregivers keeping this sentence in mind throughout caregiving and communication processes constantly will be reminded of the need for communication adaptation to be successful in relating to and interacting with recipients of their care.

Communication Problems

Several problems relating to communicating with persons with dementing illness can be predicted from the content of this previously discussed sentence. One is that of short term memory loss. Another is poor ability to concentrate. A third is extremely slowed response to stimuli, whether it be conversation or some other type of noise or input. Mother reacted very slowly to many types of inputs. For example, the telephone would ring, I would answer the phone, and about a minute or two later she recognized the phone had rung and answered it. Or, Mother and I would be having a conversation and 2-3 minutes later, or sometimes even hours later, she began communicating about the subject I presented earlier. Many caregivers confirm having seen this slow response problem in their loved ones.

Additional problems may be that of hearing difficulties, or the need for hearing aid adjustment, or the inability to read, write, or understand.

The caregiver must thoroughly understand the difficulties the person with dementia may have in understanding written and/or verbal communication. It is important for the caregiver to picture him/herself in the shoes of the person with dementia. Normal brain functioning is diminishing. It is difficult to concentrate and to remember. It seems as if the world and current environment are too confusing. Sometimes, ignoring all incoming stimuli (including anyone trying to communicate in writing or verbally) is the only way the remnants of brain cells can keep the person from losing his/her sense of self or control.

Communication Adaptation Tips

Since it is impossible for the person with dementing illness to change or adapt, it is incumbent upon those of us who are communicating with the person to adapt our communication styles and techniques to make communication effective. With an understanding of communication problems in mind, the requirements for communication to be effective are relatively logical and straight-forward in nature:

◆   Keep background noise and activities to a minimum. It is impossible for the person with dementia to concentrate on more than one thing at a time. If you want to communicate with this person, turn off music, radios, television, and other sources of noise, and try to find a private place away from groups of people.

◆   Be certain the person with dementia can hear you speak before you start to communicate. Determine if the person can hear and/or understand by asking him/her to follow a simple verbal instruction. This action will not only assure the person can hear your particular tone and loudness of voice, but will also assist you to determine the current cognitive state of the person with whom you are attempting to communicate. There can be a great deal of cognitive variability from minute to minute, hour to hour, day to day, week to week, etc. What is understood and responded to at one point in time may not be responded to at another point in time. Cognitive abilities both increase and decrease thoughout the day. Don't assume that because you get no response at one point that there will never be a response.

◆ Be certain the person with dementia has vision capabilities and can understand written communication before you attempt to communicate in writing. Determine if the person can see and/or read and understand written communication by giving the person a simple instruction written on a piece of paper.

◆ Communicate with honesty and feeling—don't attempt to beat around the bush or hide something. The person with dementia may be much more aware of what you are thinking and feeling than you know. The person with dementing illness develops a keen sensitivity to changes in tone and inflection of voice and to facial expressions and body language.

◆ Use touch to get attention and encourage the person to focus.

◆ Locate yourself so that you are at eye level in front of the person with dementing illness. Communicating from across the room, or when entering the room to the person's back or side may be very frightening to the person with dementia, and even if the person is not startled, communication will be ineffective due to the need to focus and concentrate for communication to occur.

◆ Look directly at the person and address him or her by name to get attention.

◆ Talk slowly, calmly, and deliberately. Give the person time to respond before giving up or repeating the comment or question. Remember, response time can be greatly delayed in the person with dementing illness.

- Use short sentences—five or six words in length. Wait for a response before launching into the next comment or question. Remember, the person with dementia has a great deal of difficulty in understanding long, convoluted sentences. In later stages, you may have to reduce sentences to one or two words—just subject and verb to improve comprehension and response.

- Repeat unanswered questions or comments using the exact same words. Since the person with dementia is having difficulty concentrating and has a slow response time, he/she will not be able to keep up or grasp your message if you change the wording before he/she has time to respond to your original comment or question. You may have to repeat several times before evoking a response.

- As a means of ascertaining the cognitive capacity of your loved one, frequently ask questions which cannot be answered with "yes" or "no." Open ended questions will provide you with more information about the thoughts and concerns of the person with dementia. It becomes all too easy for the person with dementia to automatically respond with "yes," or "no."

For example: Incorrect: "Did you eat this morning?"

                Correct: "What did you eat this morning?"

However, not everyone can respond to questions designed to encourage thinking. If the person with whom you are communicating is having difficulty responding to questions requiring more complex answers, or is obviously frustrated with open ended questions, you may have to resort to short questions requiring "yes" or "no" responses.

♦   When giving choices, offer only two options.

For example:	Incorrect:	"What would you like to do this morning?"
	Correct:	"Would you like to watch TV or read the paper?"

♦   Give liberal amounts of praise for all appropriately answered questions or responses.

♦   Sitting holding hands or cradling the person in the your arms communicates caring and nurturing and is a wonderful form of communication.

Remember, there can be great variability in cognitive abilities of the person with dementia throughout the day. At times, the person may be able to respond to normal conversation. At other times, the brain doesn't seem to be functioning. Therefore, checking for hearing, vision, and understanding is important each time you begin to communicate with the person with dementing illness.

Communicating on the telephone may be a good way to require focusing on a conversation. It is important, however, to keep other activities and noise in the background to a minimum so the person with dementia can focus totally on information being received on the telephone. Speaker telephones may be very effective in encouraging communication, as they do not require holding the handset at ear level, the act of which may reduce ability to concentrate on the conversation at hand.

Communication is a wonderful way for persons with dementing illness to build self-esteem and gain a sense of belongingness in this difficult world. However, caregivers and others interacting must be careful not to correct or be critical of inaccurate responses, or the act of communicating becomes a source of stress and anxiety, rather than an esteem-building activity.

Communication Subjects

Finding subjects about which to communicate can be a problem for caregivers and for friends or relatives, particularly those who visit only occasionally. Many people are so uncomfortable they stop visiting a friend or loved one with dementing illness because they feel they cannot communicate. The caregiver can be helpful in educating visitors about techniques to use as well as subjects to discuss that will bring some interaction with the person with dementing illness.

Some of the best topics to discuss are events and people from the person's past. Some people shy away from talking about past times and events, thinking this type of discussion may make the person with dementia feel sad that he/she isn't the way he used to be. In fact, persons with dementia have memory recall of early life events even in the latter stages of dementia and love to discuss treasured memories from days gone by. Be warned, however, that the person may think he/she is discussing the present. Utilizing pictures of family or friends to promote thought processes can be a very effective method of enhancing communication. Even without good vision, painting a verbal picture for the person with dementing illness can frequently bring a myriad of responses.

Events of early childhood, school, or recollection of the person's profession or occupation may be much more clear than something that happened last year, last week, or five minutes ago.

Mother, for instance, recited nursery rhymes with ease, and could still belt out her college fight song until the week before she passed away. One of her most enjoyable activities was sitting with friends or relatives, listening to music and singing along with taped musical groups such as "Sing Along With Mitch," playing on the stereo.

Caregivers mindful of communication problems of persons with dementing illness, and who take the time and possess the patience to work on communication skills, will be rewarded in all aspects of caregiving. They will be able to elicit information and responses from persons with dementia that will make caregiving considerably easier, and improve the quality of life both for the disease victims and for themselves.

6

THE ART OF CUEING—AN ESSENTIAL SKILL FOR CAREGIVERS

As the person's dementia progresses, the caregiver increasingly will be involved with coaching and behavior reinforcement. The key element to understand here is not how to tell the person what to do, but rather to lead the person down the intellectual road either verbally or in writing so that the person can more independently perform physical and intellectual functions. This technique is called cueing. A simple definition of the word *"cueing"* is prompting. Learning the art and skill of cueing, coupled with effective communication skills, is essential for all persons working with those with dementing illness.

Initiation of a cueing routine needs to occur at the first sign the person with dementia is having difficulty in performing a specific activity. If cueing routines are established in the early stages of dementing illness, the person will be able to learn the steps and maintain independent functioning longer.

Cueing can be either in the form of verbal coaching or in the form of written outlines, schedules, or instructions. The goal of cueing is to assist the person in mental thinking processes which will lead him/her to perform correct behaviors and make appropriate decisions. I have arbitrarily categorized cueing into two segments: one which describes cueing to promote independent functioning; and the other which describes cueing to promote logical thinking processes.

Cueing To Promote Independence In Performing Normal Activities

Cueing techniques work well in promoting more independent functioning in activities of daily living such as oral hygiene, bathing, and dressing.

The most essential element of appropriate cueing for independent functioning is that there be a consistent pattern which is applied by all persons interacting with the person with dementia. This consistency in application of exact steps requires that all caregivers have in writing, step by step, the procedures and methods that are being taught and/or utilized.

For example, in the case of cueing for a person who is having difficulty getting up out of a chair, the verbal cueing or coaching steps might be:

"Place hands on chair arms.

Move to the edge of the chair.

Get belly even with edge of seat.

Move feet back.

Put feet shoulder width apart.

Lean forward.

Nose over toes.

Push forward and up.

Stand up tall."

This type of specific coaching in the steps leading to accomplishment of a procedure can be utilized for all types of activities of daily living, including steps for performing oral hygiene, bathing, dressing, meal preparation, and other household tasks.

If any caregiver utilizes different words or skips any of the steps, the person with dementia will not be able to learn or relearn the appropriate steps for getting out of a chair, for example. I have experienced the rewards of working repetitively with cueing to dramatically improve physical and mental performance of persons with dementing illness.

The process of cueing initially might mean verbally coaching each step, offering praise for each completed step. Eventually, the person may be able to recall a forgotten step with an appropriately worded question or comment from the caregiver. Finally, the person will be able to remember the steps independently, or with minimal verbal coaching. Patience and repetition are the key ingredients to successful training or retraining of the brain.

Even if the person with dementia cannot remember the steps to carry out an activity after consistent cueing, and has to be verbally coached, at least the activity will be able to be performed without the physical assistance of the caregiver.

Written cueing works in the same way as verbal cueing, except, after being certain the person with dementia can **read and understand** written instructions, a card with the written cues is displayed in the appropriate place. Refer to Appendices C and D at the end of this book for sample cueing regimens.

Frequently, if cueing regimens are initiated at the very first sign of memory and/or functional problems, the regimens actually become habitual, allowing for performance of specific functions independently for a much longer period of time. Initially, the person with dementia may be able to read and follow written cueing instructions. Then as memory begins to deteriorate, simple verbal coaching from the caregiver, utilizing the written regimen, may be necessary. Finally, verbally coaching the person through each procedural step may be required.

The fact that communication and cueing skills, and the consistent application of both are the most important factors in caring for the person with dementia, dictates the pattern of caregiver scheduling. The more consistency of caregivers that can be provided, the more consistency there will be in carrying out necessary procedures and regimens. Therefore, it is better to schedule caregivers to work longer shifts to provide daily consistency, than to schedule several people working short shifts during the course of a day. Close communication among caregivers is essential to maintain consistency in behavioral cueing.

Group homes, assisted living units, and skilled nursing facilities should have specifically developed cueing schedules for all activities of daily living. These schedules must be in writing and all staff must be educated and required to use them for all residents with cognitive impairment.

The alternative to verbal and written cueing is to tell the person what to do, or worse yet, to do something for the person that he either is capable of doing, or able to be trained or coached to do him/herself. The person with dementia, who may be feeling totally inadequate (although probably not wanting to admit same), may have lowered self-esteem, and may be depressed, will only get worse if everything he/she can do is done by others. Simple actions like answering the phone or turning on the television can be major accomplishments for someone with dementing illness. Place yourself in the shoes of the person you are caring for. What would you want? I never have met anyone with dementia who didn't want to do as much as possible for him/herself, or anyone who didn't respond to behavior modification techniques of praise and reward for a job well done.

Cueing to improve independent functioning is relatively straight-forward and easy to perform. The most difficult aspect for the caregiver is breaking down behaviors into small enough steps for the person with dementia to follow. Cueing routines and schedules must be updated periodically, as the need for more detail and assistance will increase as the disease process decreases the degree of cognitive functioning. I cannot emphasize enough the importance of establishing routines early in the dementing illness process so they become somewhat habitual in nature, and will promote independence of functioning longer into the disease process.

Cueing not only will allow the person with dementia to perform many behavioral functions without physical assistance from caregivers, but also will provide a form of mental stimulation.

Caregivers need to recognize the tremendous effort required for persons with dementing illness to perform activites of daily living. Praise each step appropriately accomplished by the person with dementing illness as well as the completed task. Praising or rewarding the person will promote feelings of accomplishment and self-esteem and encourage the person to continue to perform activities of daily living.

Cueing to Promote Logical Thinking Processes or Stimulate Memory

Cueing to promote reality-oriented thinking is a real challenge to the caregiver. However, I have had a great deal of success in this area in working with a small number of persons with dementia. I will explain this type of cueing process by giving a detailed example of a situation which frequently occurred in interactions with my mother.

Mother had periods where she knew my name and knew I was her daughter. Alternately she had periods where she either knew my name, but had no idea I was related to her, or didn't know my name at all. This variability in mental functioning serves as an example of why it is so important to do some reality testing before beginning to communicate with or work with the recipient of your care. When Mother did not know me, I began a cueing process to gradually bring her to the point where she remembered who I was. This process evolved as follows (in very slow fashion). Mother's responses are italicized.

- Me: "What is my name?"
  Mother: *"I don't know."*
  Me: "That's O.K. Maybe you will think of it later."

- Me: "What is your name?"
  Mother: *"Elsie."*
  Me: "Right."

- Me: "What is your last name?"
  Mother: *"Bridges, Elsie Bridges."*
  Me: "That's right."

- Me: "Whom did you marry?"
  Mother: *"Walter Bridges."*
  Me: "Yes, very good."

- Me: "Did you have children?"
  Mother: *"Yes."*

- Me: "What were their names?"
  Mother: *"I can't remember."*
  Me: "That's O.K. Don't worry about it. You will think of their names later."

- Me: "How did you sign your Christmas cards? Walter, Elsie..."
  Mother: *"Barbara, Bruce, and Byron."*
  Me: "Right—Walter, Elsie, Barbara, Bruce, and Byron."

- Me: "Did you have any children?"
  Mother: *"Yes, Barbara, Bruce, and Byron."*
  Me: "Very good."

- Me: "What is my name?"
  Mother: *"Barbara."*

- Me: "Barbara what?"
  Mother: *"Barbara Joan Bridges."*
  Me: "Right."

- Me: "Could I be your daughter, Barbara?"
  Mother: *"Yes, you could be. I think you are."*

- Me: "I'm so glad you remember, Mother. I love you so much." (I give her a big hug).

It is very difficult to portray the feelings and tone of the conversation in writing. But, the look of relief on Mother's face when she suddenly recognized me was worth all of the painstaking effort it took on both of our parts to walk through the cueing steps to stimulate some part of her memory.

The major concept utilized in this example is to take the person back in time to points he/she might remember, and then build back up in time to the present. That is the reason I took Mother back in time to determine if she knew whom she married. Had she not had an appropriate response to that question, I would have gone farther back in time to ask about names of her parents and her siblings.

It is very important to remember that each individual with dementia responds to different types of cues. The "How do you sign your Christmas card?" question was a brainstorm of mine one day when Mother seemed to be particularly out of touch with the present. Fortunately, it worked beautifully, and subsequently, I utilized that cue on numerous occasions with continued success.

As you start this type of cueing you will have to experiment a great deal to determine what works for your loved one. Although tedious in process, the very act of working objectively with your loved one to bring some kind of rational response can be rewarding both for you, the caregiver, and for the person with dementia. Additionally, cueing places you as caregiver in a more therapeutic role, reducing some of the emotional stress of managing a loved one with dementing illness.

Again, I stress that this process takes place over time. No one with dementia can stand a bombardment of questions. You might have to stop right in the middle of cueing if you determine your loved one either cannot respond to your questions or is getting stressed by your cueing.

Some people feel this type of cueing promotes stress and frustration for the person with dementing illness. However, the people with dementia with whom I have worked are extremely pleased to be assisted to remember things that are important to them. Mother described the fright of not knowing who I was and where she was. She also described the relief when she finally knew who I was and what was happening. As I worked with Mother, I became increasingly perceptive as to when she needed cueing from me to become more comfortable. When she was having difficulty remembering or doing something of importance to her, the anxiety was visible in her eyes and on her face. She had difficulty doing anything at all, including eating, until she was more grounded and had resolved whatever was bothering her.

A note of caution is important at this juncture. The caregiver must determine if and when the person with dementing illness is capable of continuing on with this type of cueing process. There are occasional times when I determined after the first question or two, that Mother's mental state would not lend itself to cueing. However, at a later time, cueing worked well. Sometimes, if I had to stop the cueing process because I determined it was too much for her to manage, she continued the mental process herself and all of a sudden told me she knew who I was. What a delightful experience!

Additionally, it is easy to see why close family members or friends who know the person's background well can function better in this type of cueing situation. Employed caregivers simply may not have enough information to guide someone through the process to stimulate memory of past events and relationships. However, caregivers unfamiliar with past history and background may be able to stimulate memory by asking "who, what, where, and when" types of questions to probe for information assimilated in a logical fashion. Avoid "why" questions because they require too much cognitive skill to answer—they are too abstract. Institutional caregivers are advised to ask family members to provide a written life history, preferably with pictures, so caregivers will be able not only to respond to questions or comments which at times may seem to "come out of the blue," but also to communicate about subjects which may be familiar to the person with dementing illness.

By utilizing cueing concepts, hopefully, those of you in the caregiving role will be able to elicit memory responses that will enable both the person with dementia and you as a caregiver to have a more fulfilling relationship.

7

MAINTAINING PHYSICAL FUNCTIONING AND WELL-BEING

It is difficult for those of us who are dementia-free to perceive the difficulties people with dementia have in performing what should be habitual daily activities such as eating, sleeping, bathing, or dressing. What seems like a simple task to us becomes very complex for the person with dementia. Additionally, fears develop, which may prevent persons with dementia from even attempting to perform these simple and routine activities.

There are several areas of concern for the caregiver in maintaining physical functioning and well-being of the person with dementia. They will be presented in general context here, and discussed as necessary in following sections. Many of the following sections begin with "what if" questions. These questions depict actual observations I have made in caring for people with dementing illness.

Maintaining Adequate Nutrition

What if you couldn't remember when to eat, what to eat, or which meal time it is? What if you couldn't make a shopping list to buy what you needed? What if you began chewing your food, but couldn't remember to swallow, so you chewed, and chewed, and chewed? What if your sense of taste and smell were diminished so you couldn't enjoy your food? These are just a few of the nutrition problems facing the person with dementia.

Maintaining a well-balanced, nutritious diet is essential for all people, but especially important for the older adult. Frequently the person with dementia will be unable to shop for food, to prepare food, may forget to eat, or may not remember the ingredients of a well-balanced diet. The importance of adequate amounts of vitamins and minerals to maintain both physical and mental functioning is well documented.

The Food Guide Pyramid published by the U.S. Department of Agriculture is a good base for establishing nutritional requirements for the older adult. Under these guidelines, a balanced diet consists of the following servings on a daily basis:

+ 6 servings from the bread, cereal, rice and pasta group.

    One serving consists of: 1 slice of bread; 1 ounce of dry cereal; or $\frac{1}{2}$ cup cooked cereal, rice, or pasta.

+ 3 servings from the vegetable group.

One serving consists of: 1 cup of raw leafy vegetables; $\frac{1}{2}$ cup of other vegetables, cooked or chopped raw; or $\frac{3}{4}$ cup vegetable juice.

- 2 servings from the fruit group.

  One serving consists of: 1 medium apple, banana, or orange; $\frac{1}{2}$ cup chopped, cooked, or canned fruit; or $\frac{3}{4}$ cup fruit juice.

- 2 servings from the milk, yogurt, and cheese group.

  One serving consists of: 1 cup milk or yogurt; $1\frac{1}{2}$ ounces cheese; or 2 ounces of process cheese.

- 2 servings from the meat, poultry, fish, dry beans, eggs, and nuts group or a total of 5 ounces daily.

  One serving consists of 2-3 ounces of cooked lean meat, fish, or poultry.

  Note: $\frac{1}{2}$ cup of cooked dry beans, 1 egg, or 2 Tablespoons of peanut butter count as one ounce of meat.

- Fats, Oils, and Sweets group—use sparingly.

Additionally, vitamin and mineral supplements may be considered. There is a growing body of evidence supporting the use of additional supplements. Calcium deters bone loss, thereby preventing osteoporosis, a disease which can occur in both men and in women. Additional iron, found in vitamin supplements, serves to increase the oxygen carrying capacity of the blood. Some of the minor trace elements may increase mental functioning. The antioxidant vitamin group plus zinc may increase hearing, slow the progress of macular degeneration of the eyes, and may lower cholesterol. Therefore, the following supplements should be considered. Check with your family physician before utilizing supplements.

- A daily dose of therapeutic multi-vitamins.

- A daily dose of antioxidant vitamins plus zinc, labeled as vitamins and minerals for the eye.

- Calcium to make a total of 1500 mg. for women and 1200 mg. for men.

  One cup of milk contains approximately 300 mg. of calcium. One cup of yogurt contains about 375 mg. of calcium. Calcium supplements can be taken to meet the total requirements if they are not met by eating dairy products. Calcium tablets are available in 500 or 600 mg. sizes. Also, antacids containing calcium carbonate may be taken. Calcium carbonate tablets of 750 mg. contain only 300 mg. of calcium. Therefore, one would have to take four tablets daily to get 1200 mg. of calcium.

It is important that vitamin or mineral supplements be taken with meals, as they will be absorbed and utilized best if digested with food.

There may be physiological problems with chewing and/or swallowing food. As we age, taste, smell, and the amount of saliva in our mouths seem to decrease. The lack of saliva can be a very difficult problem for the person with dementia. It is sometimes difficult to ascertain whether prolonged chewing of a bite is due to the inadequate supply of liquid with which to swallow, or if the person with dementia just forgets to swallow. However, grinding or chopping foods that are not slippery in nature, or foods that require undue chewing, can greatly reduce excess chewing. Additionally, adding lots of sauces or gravies to foods makes them easier to swallow. When I prepared foods for Mother, I used lots of non-fat sour cream, yogurt, or milk to make drier foods easier to swallow.

As motor coordination deteriorates, there may be a need to obtain special utensils to enable the person with dementing illness to feed him/herself. These utensils are made for people who have had a stroke. They have handles and bends which allow the person to grip the utensil in his/her fist, rather than holding them the usual way. Utilizing special utensils may make eating much more comfortable for the person having difficulty in motor coordination of the fingers and hands.

As it becomes more difficult for the person to coordinate getting food on utensils, a plate with a large scooped edge, or one with partitions may make eating easier. These plates can be a great help to vision impaired individuals, as well.

It is not unusual for the person with dementing illness to aspirate (inhale into the lungs) liquids as they are swallowed, particularly in later stages of the disease process. The person with multi-infarct disease may be more prone to aspiration of liquids. Aspiration may be decreased by offering thicker liquids. However, if sweet, heavy liquids are aspirated, they will tend to create an environment in the lungs which is ideal for the growth of bacteria. Aspiration pneumonia may result. Thickened liquids, mostly sweet and high in calories, may lead to excessive weight gain. Therefore, I recommend that if aspiration is a common problem, you serve only clear liquids such as water, juices, broth, or tea, which will not provide an environment for the development of pneumonia if inhaled into the lungs.

Much more important than providing thickened liquids is utilizing practical techiques to prevent aspiration. Straight sided small glasses cannot be readily tipped and controlled by the person with dementing illness. Use slanted side, wide-mouth glasses. Avoid the use of straws, which invariably cause aspiration, especially in the later stages of dementia. Another important preventive technique is to allow plenty of time in the eating and drinking process. Additionally, make certain the person's head and neck are in appropriate alignment, not off to one side. Finally, recognize that the most important aspect of preventing pneumonia is the ingestion of adequate amounts of fluids to keep the lining of the bronchial tree moist and the secretions in the lungs liquid. Stimulating coughing periodically is important, as well. Simply instruct the person to "cough" occasionally.

It has long been observed that persons in later stages of dementia not only lose the ability to feed themselves, but also have increasing swallowing problems. My observations and those of others are that these problems usually occur in a more stressful dining environment. It would appear that eating in large groups, in institutional dining rooms, is too much for the person with dementia to manage. Stress from this type of stimulation creates either an action of total withdrawal resulting in the appearance of not being able to feed themselves or having the "lump in the throat" syndrome that we all experience when under a great deal of stress. One of my clients became so frightened in a noisy institutional dining environment that she refused not only to feed herself, but also to eat, resulting in massive weight loss in her first few months in a skilled nursing facility. Moving her to a more quiet small-group environment reduced her anxiety to the point that she was once again able to eat and began to regain her weight.

Any extra noise or stimulation during the dining experience, even when dining in a small group or alone can be a problem, as well. Music during dinner time may be soothing to those of us without dementia, but may provide too much stimulation and confusion for the person with cognitive impairment.

As cognitive capacity decreases, it becomes more and more important for the person with dementia not to be faced with a great assortment of food, utensils, and other items placed on the table. Varieties and assortments only cause confusion, and the person with dementing illness doesn't know where to begin. Have you ever tried to eat in an airplane? Eating off of trays is difficult for most of us. Imagine being the person with dementia who may have limited capacity to reach, may be at a table of the incorrect height, or may have difficulty with fine muscle control. Eating off a tray is nearly impossible for the person with diminished motor capacity as well as diminished mental capacity. It is also difficult to eat while sitting in an easy chair or geri-chair. Be certain the person with dementing illness is sitting in a straight backed chair with table at appropriate height to enable the eating process.

Remove any items of clutter in the eating area. Place only the foods you wish the person to consume directly in front of the person. Serve small portions so the person doesn't feel overwhelmed. It is better to have only one plate with all of the food on it, rather than several separate dishes. Remove all utensils that will not be utilized for the current food(s). Consider serving in courses, so the person only has to cope with one utensil and one plate or dish at a time. For the severely cognitively impaired person, you may have to serve only one food item on the plate at a time.

Mother declined markedly during the course of completing this book. As she declined, eating became more and more of a problem. After having several mini-strokes, she seemed to lose her ability to feed herself. Actually, she could still feed herself, but wouldn't do so without cueing to get every bite of food on the utensil, and then cueing to put the bite in her mouth. She also lost her ability to communicate verbally in phrases or sentences, but still answered questions with "yes" and "no" responses.

There is no question in my mind but what Mother knew exactly what I was asking her to do or what questions I was asking. She simply could not respond, even though she understood perfectly. I determined that she did want to eat—her not eating was not an attempt to indicate she had had enough of this whole situation. She still was able to express when she had had enough food. She simply would stop swallowing, and when I asked her if she was full, she would answer, "yes." Sometimes she ate without cueing at all, and other times she needed total cueing to feed herself. She was able to communicate to me that she knew food was in front of her when she was reminded, but after taking one bite she forgot and thought about other things. It was very frustrating to her that her food was sitting and getting cold. She wanted to be reminded when she was not eating, and reminded to take each bite if necessary. She despised being fed. It made her feel like she was a "little baby." I never did feed her, rather I would place the food on the utensil and assist her in guiding the food to her mouth.

We have learned that we should serve hot foods hot and cold foods cold. The person with dementing illness, however, may not be able to tolerate very hot or very cold foods. It has been my observation that beverages and other hot foods, even if they feel lukewarm to me, are too hot for someone with dementia. Additionally, very cold foods may be too cool. Serve fruits and other refrigerated items at room temperature. Carefully check hot foods before they are served. Ascertain from the person with dementia the temperature at which food feels comfortable for him/her to eat.

Maintaining a set meal schedule is important not only for optimal physical functioning of the older adult, but also for assisting with memory retention and promotion of independence. Additionally, many potential bowel and bladder functioning problems can be prevented by establishing consistent meal times.

Maintaining an appropriate level of weight for the size and stature of the person is important as well. Caregivers should record monthly weights, taken before breakfast at the same time each month, to adequately assess weight maintenance. Overweight people will have more difficulty with physical functioning as their cognitive abilities diminish. Therefore, decreasing food amounts and encouraging exercise with the goal of promoting gradual weight loss is important for the overweight person with dementing illness.

Maintaining adequate weight is equally important. An underweight person must be given frequent snacks, preferably nutritious ones, but if the person continues to be underweight, high calorie and high fat snacks are essential. Hyperactivity in the more agitated person with dementia contributes greatly to weight loss. In this situation, not only should hourly snacks be provided, but also more sedate activities should be utilized to minimize weight loss from too much activity.

Continuing weight loss in the presence of adequate nutrition and high calorie snacks should be reported to a physician, as some other physical disease may be the cause.

Maintaining Adequate Fluid Intake

What if you couldn't tell when you were thirsty? What if you couldn't remember if and when you last had anything to drink?

Maintaining an adequate degree of hydration becomes increasingly difficult for the person with dementia. Not only does the person forget to drink, but also, his/her sensation of thirst may be diminished. As persons age, their joints, including their neck joints become less flexible. Therefore, it becomes very difficult for the older person to tip his/her head back far enough to get liquids out of a straight edged or small glass. When offering liquids, do so in an exaggeratedly slanted side, wide-mouth glass or cup. Try utilizing a straw if aspiration isn't a problem. Additionally, it is very difficult for the aging person to hold a cup with a small handle which accommodates only a finger or two. Provide a cup with a large handle which can be grabbed between the thumb and many fingers.

Adequate fluid levels are essential for all body functions, including: elimination (bowel and bladder); respiratory; kidney; liver; cardiac; and brain. Dehydration may lead to recurrent urinary tract infections, low blood pressure, fainting, constipation, or recurrent respiratory infections. Fluid monitoring is an essential role of the caregiver. One easy way to be alert to the degree of hydration is to check the color of the person's urine. Urine should be a pale, straw, light yellow color. If urine is golden, or a concentrated yellow, the person is underhydrated.

Adequate fluid intake for most adults is around two quarts of liquids per day (approximately eight full 8-ounce glasses). More than 2 quarts of fluid may be required for persons living in an extremely hot or dry climate or for persons undergoing a lot of physical activity. The type of fluid consumed is equally as important as the amount.

Fluids to minimize or avoid are as follows:

♦   Coffee—the caffeine in coffee may act as a stimulant, increasing anxiety and confusion, may react with other medications the person is taking, and even if coffee is decaffeinated, it is diuretic in nature, causing the tendency toward dehydration.

♦   Carbonated beverages which are caffeinated have the same effect as coffee.

♦   Strong tea may contain equally as much caffeine as a cup of coffee. Herbal and decaffeinated teas in moderation are fine.

♦   Alcohol not only is dehydrating, but also has the effect of decreasing mental functioning—a particular problem with the person with dementia. Additionally, alcohol can react with other prescribed medications, causing mental incapacitation or impairment of physical functioning. If alcohol is requested, it should be consumed in extreme moderation (one drink) and in very dilute form. Non-alcoholic beers and wines are now available, which are safe in moderation and taste good to the person with dementing illness.

Fluids to encourage are juices and water.

Timing of fluid intake is important, as well. Many persons with dementia have difficulty with bladder control, especially when sleeping at night. Therefore, the two quarts of fluid should be consumed throughout the day, but minimized after the last meal in the evening. Fluids should be spaced throughout the day between meals. It is impossible for any person to drink all required fluids with the usual three major meals.

If the person with dementia does not drink willingly, it may be a problem of approach of the caregiver. Consider the following caregiver approaches to attempting to get someone to drink:

◆ "Honey, would you like something to drink?"

◆ "It's time for you to drink something. Would you like water or apple juice?"

◆ "Your urine is too dark. You need to drink. Would you like orange juice or cranberry juice?"

The first approach is social and pleasant, but it is not therapeutic in nature. The response of someone who does not like to drink will probably be "no." The last two approaches, one more clinical than the other, set an expectation that the person should drink, but does so in a matter of fact, non-demanding way. Note, the person is given a choice, creating a feeling of participation in the decision making process. If a change in approach does not work, never force someone to drink. Simply try at a later time. Remember, scheduling fluid intake times as a part of the routine will encourage drinking.

Maintaining Bowel and Bladder Functions

What if you couldn't tell if you had to urinate or have a bowel movement? What if you went into the bathroom, but forgot to remove your clothing before urinating? What if you had an accident in your clothes and you either didn't recognize you had a problem, or didn't know what to do about your soiled clothes?

The person with dementing illness may have increasing difficulties with bowel and bladder functioning as the disease process progresses. Therefore, it is extremely important to establish bowel and bladder routines at the very beginning of the disease process. Establishing these routines can prevent and/or delay malfunction of these elimination systems. Monitoring frequency and character of bowel and bladder evacuations is an essential role of the caregiver.

Important to these elimination functions is the consumption of adequate fluids as described in the above section. Additionally, eating large amounts of high fiber content foods, such as whole grains, fruits, and vegetables, will aid bowel functioning. Frequently persons with dementia have decreased speed of intestinal motility, making the food stay in the intestines longer, causing constipation. Prunes and prune juice are especially helpful to the older person, as they increase the speed with which contents move through the intestines. Routine consumption of over-the-counter fiber capsules may be of help. **Maintaining adequate fluid intake is extremely important if fiber capsules are consumed.**

Loss of sensation of needing to have a bowel movement or needing to urinate may be a problem for the person with dementing illness. This loss of sensation may lead to constipation from not evacuating the bowel, or to bowel or bladder incontinence with many resultant problems. A schedule for bowel and bladder evacuation is essential, not only for delaying such problems, but also for minimizing these problems if they occur.

◆   Bowel evacuation scheduling and monitoring.

Determining past bowel patterns and habits is essential to setting up a bowel evacuation schedule. However, a set time daily to evacuate bowels will be consistent with most people's bowel habits. This time is usually after breakfast. If no bowel movement occurs after breakfast, the person should be encouraged to try again after each meal, until a bowel movement occurs. As muscle tone and/or mental capacity decrease, it may be necessary for the caregiver to stay with the person with dementia, either to provide verbal coaching to remember to push, or to utilize abdominal support with gentle pressure on the lower abdomen while instructing the person to take a deep breath and push.

If more than one caregiver is involved, it is important to record the date, time, amount, and character of bowel movements to be certain bowels are functioning normally. A single caregiver can usually track bowel movements without written records. Be particularly mindful of any change of bowel movements to a black or tarry consistency. This color change could indicate bleeding from the gastrointestinal tract, and should be reported to a physician immediately.

It is important that activities be scheduled around bowel and bladder evacuation schedules, rather than vice versa.

♦   Bladder evacuation scheduling and monitoring.

Urinary tract problems are frequent with older adults. Poor fluid intake, poor muscle tone, lack of sensation of needing to urinate all contribute to problems. Urinary tract infections can be prevalent in both sexes, but particularly in females. An enlarged prostate gland in males may cause partial blockage of the urinary tract, leading to a feeling of always having to urinate, bladder spasms, and lack of bladder control (incontinence). Urinary tract infections may cause the same symptoms. Additionally, the continual pressure or back up of urine with an enlarged prostate blockage can cause irreversible renal hypertension, leading to severe kidney damage.

The person with dementing illness may be accused of exposing himself or herself or trying to undress in public, when in actuality, he or she may have a tremendous sensation of having to urinate which takes precedence over any social mores. The person with dementia may not be able to communicate or determine the nature of the problem. Therefore, the caregiver becomes the eyes, ears, and nose, and the logically thinking person relative to bladder functioning.

Persons with symptoms of frequently needing to urinate, frequently going into the bathroom, the tendency to attempt to urinate in public, incontinence, or evidence of cloudy, strong smelling, or bloody urine should be evaluated by a urologist.

Bladder problems, with resulting discomfort may be so severe that they prevent the person from focusing on other situations and may lead to agitation and frustration. Frequently the person with dementia is not able to verbalize the basis of the discomfort. Caregiver observations are crucial in evaluating bladder problems. All available medical action should be taken to correct the situation causing bladder discomfort and/or incontinence, to reduce agitation and general discomfort, as well as to prevent embarrassing situations for the person with dementing illness.

All too often persons with dementia are labeled as being "incontinent," when in actuality, they only need more frequent toileting and a bladder emptying schedule to remain dry. Wearing diapers or pads is embarrassing and humiliating for the person with dementing illness, especially if he/she is able to control his/her bladder, but not able to request or get toileting assistance frequently enough to stay dry. If correcting a medical problem or being diligent about maintaining bladder or bowel training schedules prevents or delays the use of diapers or other incontinent products, every attempt should be made by the caregiver to do so.

Determining past toileting frequency is the first step in developing a bladder emptying schedule. Toileting on a set schedule can delay and/or prevent bladder incontinence. Bladder evacuation scheduling can lead to increased bladder muscle tone and improved functioning. Usually, a schedule of every two hours will be adequate. However, if the person has a small bladder, has an enlarged prostate gland, or has an infection or some other bladder problem, hourly toileting may be required to keep the person from having bladder spasms, and/or incontinence. The caregiver can have major influence in not only preventing potential bladder problems, but also in preventing the physical discomfort, and the emotional and personal degradation which goes with them.

It is especially important for the person with partial or total incontinence to be toileted according to a schedule to retrain and/or regain bladder muscle control. If you are just initiating a bladder training program with a person having difficulty with bladder control, start with hourly toileting during the day. Gradually increase the amount of time between toileting over a period of several weeks until reaching a schedule of every 2 hours. Do not neglect toileting at night. Initially try every 2-3 hours. It is possible that the person with dementia can be kept totally dry during the day with frequent toileting, but not during the night when the person is sleeping. It will take up to three months of diligent scheduling of bladder emptying to begin to see control in someone who has been "incontinent."

It is very difficult for family caregivers to reach an adequate balance between needing sleep themselves, toileting their loved ones, and allowing enough time between toileting episodes for their loved ones with dementia to get adequate sleep, as well. I strongly encourage caregivers to toilet their loved ones at least twice during a typical eight hour night. Leaving someone in a urine saturated bed, or in urine saturated diapers not only creates the potential for infections and skin breakdown, but also is tremendously humiliating for the person with dementing illness. Adequate emptying of the bladder cannot occur in a recumbent position. Poor emptying contributes to the possibility of infection. Therefore, it is essential to get the person in a sitting or standing position to urinate.

Placing a commode or urinal at the bedside will minimize the time and effort needed for nighttime toileting, and prevent both the caregiver and person with dementia from becoming awakened by bright lights and the hassle of assisting someone to the bathroom. Frequently commodes placed adjacent to the head of the bed, facing toward the foot of the bed, can be utilized without caregiver assistance. The person simply slides from the position in bed to the immediately available commode at the side of the bed.

If you have diligently tried and maintained a bladder training program for two to three months and have checked with a urologist to determine there is no treatable cause, and the person with dementia is still having problems with bladder control, you will have to provide products to keep the person dry. Fortunately, there are many products available that did not exist even a couple of years ago. Both disposable products and reusable or launderable products are available. Reusable products, of course, are more environmentally sound. Reusable products usually are available only at medical supply stores. Some baby diaper services provide adult diapers, as well. Many discount stores provide these products in larger quantities at a markedly reduced price.

Products for daytime use range from full pant diapers to all weights of small pads to insert in under garments. I would encourage you to use the smallest and most comfortable product available which will still keep the person under your care from having any embarrassing accidents. However, the use of products requiring the negotiation of elastic straps or buttons is nearly impossible for the person with dementing illness. If adult diapers or pads are worn, they must be changed when damp to prevent skin excoriation. Diapers must be changed minimally every two hours, (if damp), with the genital area washed with mild soap and water before a new diaper is applied. Adult-sized packaged wipes for washing the genital area now are available. However, nothing substitutes for occasional cleaning with warm soapy water.

If the person with dementing illness is incontinent during the day, necessitating the use of diapers or heavy pads, it is advisable to leave the genital area uncovered at night to prevent skin problems. This will necessitate the use of some sort of pad to protect the linens and mattress from becoming soiled during the night.

Two types of bed pads are available that are both comfortable and absorbent of urine. Medical supply stores carry very absorbent cloth pads with plastic sandwiched in the middle to protect the bed. They have non-skid surfaces on the side that is toward the bed. They absorb large volumes of urine and can be supplemented with additional specially designed felt pads cut the same size as the protective pad. They launder with ease and last a long time. Additionally, disposable pads are available. These come in all prices and weights for varying absorbency.

For additional protection of a home mattress, medical supply stores carry fitted plastic mattress covers. I recommend these covers for added protection. An alternative is to cover the mattress with overlapping small disposable pads. Infant and toddler size rubber or vinyl sheets simply are not absorbent enough for adults, and generally are not a satisfactory means of protection.

There are laundry detergent products on the market designed for use with baby diapers or urine soiled clothing. These products are very helpful in eliminating odor from urine soiled linens. I suggest you double wash these items. I generally use the special products for a soak cycle, and then wash them in regular laundry detergent for the complete wash. If linens or clothing are soiled with feces, they definitely need a soak cycle, and usually more than one complete wash cycle to eliminate odors.

Remember, latex gloves, (not vinyl), must be worn when assisting the person with urine or feces stained clothing or diapers to prevent spread of disease. Be certain both the person with dementing illness and the caregiver wash hands thoroughly after toileting.

Maintaining Adequate Sleep

What if you went to bed and didn't know if it was nighttime or daytime? What if you woke up from a nap in the afternoon, and thought it was time for breakfast? What if you became frightened or lost when in a darkened room?

There are numerous causes for sleeplessness. These include: discomfort or pain; environmental causes, such as being too warm or too cold; medications; depression; too little activity during the day; use of stimulants such as coffee; hunger; and stress. Some persons may have disease-caused delusions or hallucinations. If the person is napping a lot during the day, sleep will be difficult during the night.

The most important role of the caregiver in promoting sleep is to determine what is causing the person to be unable to sleep. Think of all of the reasons you may have difficulty in sleeping and determine if any of your reasons may be the cause. Question the person with dementing illness. If the person is up and wandering at night, determine if he/she is looking for the bathroom, too warm, hungry, or is up for some other reason. Try to correct or compensate for the problem. Do not forget the importance of scheduled nighttime toileting. Scheduled toileting a couple of times during the night may assist in preventing a great deal of nighttime restlessness.

Persons with dementia frequently become more disoriented after dark or when awakening. Fear and agitation may lead to restlessness and lack of sleep. In the evening when it begins to get dark, be certain there is very bright artificial lighting to simulate daytime prior to retiring. Leaving a night-light on in the bedroom may be of help. Placing arrows on the walls or on the floor leading to the bathroom and labeling the bathroom door in big bold print may allow the person with dementia to get to the bathroom at night with minimal assistance. As mentioned previously, an even more effective technique for dealing with toileting at night is to place a commode at the bedside. Men may wish to utilize a urinal at the bedside. Be certain the commode is stable and is adjusted to fit so the person's feet sit flat on the floor. Sitting on a commode with feet dangling in the breeze is not only uncomfortable, but also a deterrent to appropriate emptying of the bladder. I utilized sand bags tied to each commode leg to make the commode completely safe for Mother to slide over onto it without fear of tipping or falling.

Recent sleep research has shown that the myth that older people need less sleep is incorrect. Studies show that older people need eight to ten hours of sleep per day for the highest level of mental and physical functioning. However, it may be difficult for the person with dementia to sleep in long blocks of time. Therefore, short rest periods during the day may be essential.

The more uninterrupted sleep a person can sustain, the more beneficial the sleep time. This concept should be considered when scheduling re-positioning or changing of wet bedding or clothing during the night. Additionally, even though the person may have to be toileted or changed during the night, turning on bright lights should be avoided to maximize the person's ability to get back to sleep. Of course, a safe level of light must be maintained to avoid accidents or injury.

Maintaining Oral Hygiene

What if you looked in the medicine cabinet and didn't know whether to brush your teeth with shaving cream or with toothpaste? What if you thought your colorful mouthwash was a beverage? What if, when brushing your teeth, you couldn't remember to brush all tooth surfaces, so you just brushed a couple of teeth and then quit, thinking you had done a good job? What if you couldn't remember to brush your teeth at all? What if you thought your razor was for brushing your teeth?

As a person ages, physiological changes occur in the mouth which require much more effective oral hygiene to prevent both tooth decay and gum disease. The major changes are chemical in nature, with the body not secreting the concentration of enzymes which aid in the beginning digestion of food in the mouth. Additionally, many older adults secrete very little saliva, a problem which not only leads to tooth decay, but also difficulty in chewing and swallowing of food.

Persons with dementia may be perfectly competent and reliable to brush their teeth well earlier in the disease process. However, as mental functions decrease, supervision and cueing may be necessary to be certain oral hygiene is thorough. Initially, if the person can read, written cueing may be adequate. However, eventually, verbal cueing and coaching will be essential. Prevention of tooth loss and/or decay is an important role for the caregiver. Adapting to dentures is extremely difficult for the person with dementing illness.

It is very frightening to the person with dementia to have someone else attempt to perform oral hygiene. Most of us dislike going to the dentist or dental hygienist and having someone else work in our mouths. Imagine how you would feel if you could not determine why someone was trying to get into your mouth. Therefore early cueing and training to assist the person to perform oral hygiene independently, or with minimal coaching, will prevent a great deal of stress both for the person with dementing illness and for the caregiver.

Although many products such as antiplaque rinses and toothpastes have been developed, the most important part of oral hygiene in the older adult is removal of remaining food on the teeth immediately after ingestion of food. I strongly recommend use of one of the rechargeable battery operated plaque remover toothbrushes. More effective brushing occurs in a shorter time with these instruments.

Generally, good oral hygiene for persons with some or all of their own teeth incorporates the following procedure after ingestion of food (or at least after the three major meals):

• Rinse mouth with water or antiplaque rinse.

• Utilize stimudents (dental toothpicks) between all teeth to loosen food particles and massage the gums.

• Thoroughly brush all tooth surfaces with **small** amount of toothpaste.

- Rinse mouth thoroughly with water.

- Rinse mouth with fluoride mouthwash.

Once a day, teeth should be flossed, **preferably before retiring at night**, but only if the person with dementia will either perform this procedure him/herself or allow the caregiver to floss without a battle.

Persons with dentures generally need to rinse their mouths thoroughly with water and a mouthwash after eating. They may need to remove dentures to facilitate removal of food particles which lodge under the dentures. Dentures should be removed at night for thorough cleaning and soaking in a denture solution or plain water.

Maintaining Healthy Skin

The aging process also affects the skin in the older adult. Skin tends to become more like tissue paper and can tear and bruise extremely easily. Additionally, dry skin is a common problem as we age.

The major role of the caregiver is in prevention of skin problems. Daily inspection of the skin is essential to be certain problems are not developing. Inspection is most easily accomplished following a bath or at bedtime when the person is undressing. Genital area inspection is more important in females, but also necessary for males, particularly those with the problem of incontinence. If repeated bruises occur in the same place, try to determine the source of the bruise. Perhaps furniture has to be rearranged, or a sharp table corner covered.

The following suggestions will improve skin condition and/or assist in healing if a problem develops:

- Make certain nutrition and fluid intake are adequate.

- Utilize a minimal amount of soap—if soap is used, use bar soap that contains $\frac{1}{4}$ moisturizing cream, a soap frequently recommended by dermatologists. Moisturizing shower or bath gels may be utilized, as well.

- Use liberal amounts of lotion over the entire body after bathing. You will find that most lotions contain water as the most prevalent ingredient (listed first on the label). Choose any lotion that lists oil or lanolin oil as the **first** ingredient on the label.

- If a shallow skin tear occurs, utilize a small amount of antibiotic ointment and cover with one of the second skin transparent types or bioclusive types of dressings, which remain on the skin until it is healed. These dressings should always be available for immediate use by the caregiver.

- The person with incontinence should not wear diapers at night. Rather, pads should be utilized on the bed, and the skin left open to the air. If redness or rash occurs in the genital areas be particularly diligent about keeping this area clean. Medicated diaper ointments found in the infant sections of drug stores or health food stores are excellent barriers to urine and diarrheal stools, and promote rapid healing as well as immediate relief from soreness or reddened and excoriated skin in the genital areas. Different brands seem to work better on some people than on others. Therefore, try several brands to attempt to find the particular ointment which reduces soreness and promotes healing most rapidly. Of course, skin must be gently washed with soap and water prior to application of any ointment.

The development of pressure sores can occur very quickly in the older adult. Frequent changes of position, hourly during the day, and every two hours at night, can prevent these difficult-to-heal sores. It is important for persons confined to chairs to sit on a semi-hard surface rather than a very soft surface or sling seat which may be found in a wheelchair. Sitting on a more solid surface allows for some movement on the seat to reduce pressure on certain points. Sitting on a sling or very soft seat promotes continuous, unrelieved pressure on all areas of the buttocks. Wheelchairs can be fitted with memory foam solid chair seats which are excellent for prevention of pressure sores. Other items which are less effective are "egg crate" cushions, water cushions, and gel cushions. These items range in price from inexpensive to very expensive.

Moving and changing of position every two hours while reclining is essential if pressure points on hips or buttocks are a problem. Additionally, either an "egg crate" mattress pad, a sheepskin mattress pad, or, if the problem is severe, an alternating pressure air mattress contribute not only to comfort, but also to prevention and/or healing of pressure sores.

Assisting with Bathing

Bathing is a simple task. Right? But what if you are afraid of falling in the shower or tub, or you can't remember whether or not you already bathed today, yesterday, or last week. What if you are afraid of getting burned by water that is too hot? What if you can't remember how to adjust the water temperature with these "new-fangled" faucets? What if you are depressed and don't give a darn about hygiene? These are just a few of the problems that people with dementing illness may present when attempting to bathe, or for that matter, when refusing to bathe.

Caregivers need to do every thing possible to make bathing a pleasant and relaxing experience. Mother liked to soak in a tub with bubble bath and a little yellow rubber duck. This was her most relaxed time of day. Your loved one may find music to be relaxing while bathing. Determine the person's bathing likes and dislikes pre-dementia. Did the person shower or tub bathe? Bath time, by the way, is the easiest time for the caregiver to inspect the skin for redness, sores, rashes, or bruises.

It is important to determine the origin of bathing problems. Make corrections for safety. If the water is too hot, adjust the thermostat on the hot water heater. Place non-skid strips in the shower or tub bottom. Place grab bars for hands in the shower stall or tub enclosure. If the person with dementia simply does not remember to bathe, use written or verbal cueing to assist the memory process. Sometimes hair washing can be very frightening for the person with dementia. It may be appropriate to separate hair washing from bathing if this is the problem.

My experiences with water temperatures and persons with dementia is that they do not tolerate either very warm or very cold water. Other caregivers in the Alzheimer's support group which I facilitate confirm this observation. Water temperatures that felt luke warm to me, felt too hot for Mother. Be certain the person with dementing illness tests the water with a hand before entering a shower or tub with water which you have adjusted to your own temperature tastes.

Be certain the room is a comfortable temperature—usually very warm for the older person. Provide for privacy and adequate lighting. If the person is modest and needs the assistance of a caregiver, cover whatever you can with a towel while bathing. If the person is objecting to bathing, give the person some choices, such as bathing or showering. Do not get into an argumentative situation. Prepare the room and materials in advance, or set them out in order of use for the person with dementia to use him/herself. Purchase a hand-held shower wand either for hair washing or for carefully placed showering to prevent the person having to be sprayed from head down. Suggest an enjoyable activity which can occur after the bath is finished.

Encourage the person to do as much of the bath or hair washing as is possible. Assist only when needed. The genital areas are the most important to bathe to prevent skin breakdown. If the person can get in and out of the tub either with assistance or without, a tub bath should be encouraged. This will provide relaxation as well as do the best job of cleaning the genital areas.

Be certain the person is thoroughly dry after bathing. Again, the genital areas are the most important. Additionally, drying between the toes and around the feet are important to prevent fungus diseases such as "Athlete's Foot."

Assisting with Dressing

It is difficult to conceive of a simple task such as dressing being very complicated. But what if you can't distinguish dirty from clean clothes? What if you can't remember where your clothes are? What if you can't remember the sequence in which to dress? What if you can't remember whether you are getting dressed or undressed? Dressing can be a major obstacle for persons with dementing illness. The task of dressing is quite complicated. Just try to break the act of dressing down into small little steps.

Therefore, it is very important to have a neat and orderly environment for dressing. Room temperature must be comfortable. Privacy must be provided. Written cueing schedules and labels on drawers in large writing may be of assistance. A written list of clothing to put on, numbered in the order in which the items are utilized may work, as well. If the person can't read and understand, paste up clothing pictures in order of dressing. Another technique, which may work, is for the caregiver to set clothes out on the bed or somewhere where they can be placed and numbered for each of the dressing steps. For example #1 might be panties; #2 bra; #3 a blouse, etc.

Clothing may have to be adapted or changed due to decrease in fine motor coordination of the person with dementing illness. Buttons and zippers may be too difficult to manage. Vision may be poor making detailed clothing difficult to utilize. The use of pull-on fleece outfits can be very comfortable for the person with dementia. These garments are zipperless, buttonless, and very soft and comfortable. Many of these outfits made for women are very attractive, as well. If your loved one is adamant about wearing specific items of clothing with unmanageable zippers and buttons, replacing them with velcro may be a solution. Additionally, some catalogs and medical clothing stores cater to the person with finger coordination difficulties, providing attractive clothing lines adapted for ease of dressing.

As physical deterioration increases during the disease process, it will be necessary to pay particular attention to footware that will stay in place and be non-skid in nature. Comfort as well as stability are important. Good walking shoes, preferably with ties, will be the most safe and most comfortable. Slippers must be non-skid and shoe type rather than scuff type that require more coordination when walking.

When finished with bathing and dressing, have the person look in the mirror and see how he/she looks. Encourage the person to apply scents or don jewelry to complete the look. Offer praise for appearing "handsome" or "pretty." Offer praise as a reward for a job well done. The process of bathing and dressing can be very tiring for the person with dementing illness. It may be necessary to schedule a more sedate and relaxing activity or even a rest after dressing to allow for recuperation from fatigue.

Maintaining Healthy Fingernails and Toenails

Fingernails and toenails must be maintained in good condition Weekly manicures which include nail filing and applying lotions and cuticle oils usually must be provided by the caregiver, as the person with dementia frequently has visual problems as well as diminished finger coordination skills, making it impossible to maintain adequate nail care.

Daily care includes pushing back cuticles of both toenails and fingernails with a towel when drying after a shower or bath. Fungus infections are more prevalent, particularly on feet of older adults. Usually, foot fungus infections can be prevented with meticulous drying between toes and around nails following bathing. Additionally, if shoes and socks become wet, they should be changed immediately. However, if fungal infections do occur, one of the over-the-counter anti-fungal preparations can be applied twice daily to **clean, dry feet.** Application of anti-fungal powders will assist in keeping feet dry and will ease the process of pulling on socks.

Manicures and pedicures should be performed weekly, either after a five minute soaking in water or after a shower or bath. Application of cuticle removers and gentle pushing back of the cuticle is effective in preventing hangnails, which might become infected. Cuticles generally should not be clipped, to minimize the potential for infection. Filing of nails with a diamond type of file is usually safer than clipping with a nail clippers. If nails are infected with fungus, use separate files and/or clippers for fingernails and toenails. Clean instruments between each manicure and pedicure and soak them in a solution of alcohol after use. Many women benefit psychologically from the application of nail polish.

If the person's nails are too difficult to file or clip, or the person has evidence of corns, calluses, or persistent fungal infections, the consultation and assistance of a podiatrist is advised. Many local senior centers offer foot care at a reduced price on a pre-scheduled basis.

A weekly manicure and pedicure must be included on the written plan of care. One additional benefit of manicuring nails is the touching, relaxation, and stress reduction for the person with dementia.

Maintaining Visual and Auditory Aids

The aging adult may wear glasses and/or hearing aids, and frequently cannot see adequately or hear appropriately without them. Many times, this writer has observed persons who have been labeled as unable to understand due to disease processes, only to find that the problem is ineffective hearing. A major caregiver role is in seeing that hearing aids are worn, and that they are clean and maintained appropriately. Frequent inspection of eye glasses and cleaning when hazy is necessary. The person with dementing illness may not be able to determine that glasses need cleaning. Scratched glasses, or glasses that won't stay in place need to be replaced, repaired, or adjusted.

Hearing aids should always be removed and turned off at night, preferably with the battery compartment left open to air. This is a good time to inspect aids for dirt and wax. They cannot be immersed in water, but brushes and air cleaners are available to assist in keeping them clean. Hearing aids with over-the-ear receivers have tubes that harden with age. These need to be replaced periodically by a hearing aid specialist, usually at least anually—preferably every six months.

Hearing aid batteries usually need to be changed every two weeks in aids which are worn every day. The caregiver must check hearing aids daily, or any time the person seems to be having difficulty in hearing, as the person with dementia may not be aware enough to determine hearing aid problems. Most hearing aid volumes can be adjusted, once in the ear, by turning the volume completely down, and then gradually turning it up until there is a little squeal when the caregiver or the wearer cups his/her hand over the ear. Too low a volume renders the hearing aid ineffective. Too high a volume is extremely irritating to the wearer and potentially damaging to the ear. It is important for persons wearing hearing aids to have a "hearing aid compatible telephone." These phones are readily available at major telephone stores.

Persons wearing hearing aids should be seen and evaluated by an otolaryngologist or otologist annually, if for no other reason than to have excess wax, which has a tendency to build up in the ear behind hearing aids, removed from the ear canal. Additionally, persons wearing eyeglasses should by evaluated annually by an opthamologist to provide for early diagnosis and treatment of disease conditions which may be affecting eye sight, or the need to change the eyeglass prescription.

Maintaining Appropriate Posture and Alignment

What if you were off balance and falling and you thought you were perfectly positioned?

Frequently, the person with dementia has difficulty with positioning and spatial concepts. Left and right, front and back, and other directions may become confused. The person may feel balanced and centered both standing and while sitting, yet be entirely off balance or tilted while standing and crooked in bed or the chair while sitting. It is important for the caregiver to cue for correct posture and alignment for standing, sitting, or lying in bed. Incorrect posture can lead to falls, poor muscle tone and functioning, or potential injury to muscles and/or joints when changing position.

• Maintaining posture while standing and walking

The most frequent upright postural problem is the tendency to lean too far forward, especially with the upper body (head, neck, and chest), creating the potential for a forward fall. Caregivers can have the person back up to a wall to get a sense of correct posture. Also, asking the person to look at himself in a full length mirror will lead to correction of posture, providing there are no vision problems. **The caregiver must cue the person to be in a balanced standing position with upright posture before allowing movement such as walking. Before assisting with movement, allow enough time for the person to get his/her balance and be upright.**

An additional common problem is to walk and stand with feet too close together, causing balance problems. Feet placed too close together, in effect, cause the body to be like a triangle balancing on its point. Placing the feet shoulder width apart will broaden the base of the body (triangle) and promote better balance and posture. Continual cueing may be essential to correct this dangerous problem.

Whenever the caregiver sees the person with dementia off balance or out of alignment, whether walking, sitting, or lying in bed, it is important to cue the person to become straight. Continuous sitting at a tilt, or lying crooked in bed can lead to a permanent decrease in joint mobility and to muscle shortening, which will, over time cause tremendous mobility difficulties. Someone who constantly stands or sits with his/her head tilted to the same side, for example, will have difficulty in straightening the head, therefore, making it difficult to swallow and eventually, even to breath.

When standing or walking, the view from the side should be one of a vertical line extending from the ear to the shoulder to the hip bone to the ankle bone. When the head is too far forward, the buttocks too far backward, or the abdomen too far forward, the body center of gravity is changed, making balance more difficult and potential for falls greater.

◆   Maintaining posture while sitting

The person with dementing illness must always be cued to sit with his/her buttocks against the chair back. If the chair seat is too deep (the hip to knee distance is too short to scoot completely back in the chair), provide a cushion behind the person to support the entire back. Additionally, the chair must always be low enough for the person's feet to be flat on the floor when sitting. Dangling feet lead to circulatory problems due to pressure on the vessels in the back of the legs, in addition to the discomfort.

The chair type may need to be changed as the person with dementia finds it more difficult to get out of the chair. It is important to maintain all possible muscle function by providing a chair appropriate to the level of physical functioning. Whereas a rocker or swivel chair may have been comfortable and functional previously, the person with dementing illness will have an increasing need for a stable chair to allow for independent functioning. It is far better to provide a chair the person can get out of him/herself than to have to continually assist the person out of the chair. Many major muscle groups are utilized and strengthened when getting into and out of a chair. Furthermore, in trying to get out of an unstable chair, the person may lose his/her balance, fall, or strain a muscle, causing injury.

The best chair for a person looking unsteady or having a difficult time getting up from a sitting to a standing position is one with a fairly firm seat, having chair arms that go to the front edge of the seat. The back should be fairly straight or slanted back only slightly and should not be "barrel shaped." Barrel shaped chairs promote a sagging chest and shoulders which roll forward, leading to an irreversible postural problem, difficulty in breathing, and a tendency to lose one's balance when standing and walking. The chair seat should be at a height that will allow the person's feet to be flat on the floor with his/her knees approximately one inch above the hip bone. There should be a slight slope downward from the knees to the hips. Additionally, the depth of the chair seat from front to back, should be such that with the person's buttocks completely at the back of the chair, there will be about a one inch gap between the chair and the back of the knee joint. Chairs with casters or swivels must be avoided for safety reasons.

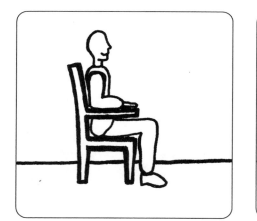

Correctly Fitting
Chair

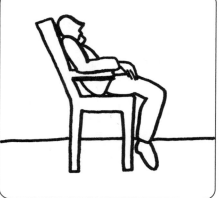

Incorrectly Fitting
Chair

Wheel chairs must be measured and fitted to the person's dimensions by an expert who knows how to fit chairs. In addition to the above mentioned factors, it is important to have flexibility in positioning of a wheel chair. Feet should be flat on the floor when sitting upright. Foot rests should be provided for long distance transportation only. The person should be able to propel the wheel chair with his/her feet to assist in maintaining muscle tone of the legs. Chair arm heights should be adjustable for varying needs, to go under a table top, for example.

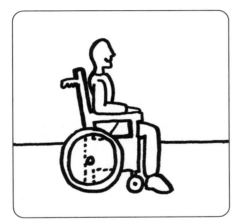

| Correctly Fitting Wheel Chair | Incorrectly Fitting Wheel Chair |

I discourage the use of both "geri chairs" and motorized re-cliners. Both of these chairs minimize self-movement and increase the speed of muscle decline. Geri chairs place a great deal of stress on the back in the semi-recumbent and recumbent positions. Motorized recliners are usually very large in structure—too large for most people, causing a great deal of discomfort and stress on the back, as well as muscle mass decline. The person with dementing illness will not be able to verbalize discomfort from an inappropriately fitting chair.

◆   Maintaining posture when reclining

Maintaining appropriate posture while lying in bed is important, as well. Generally, the recommended position in bed is
lying on one's side. Lying on the back or the stomach puts a
great deal of stress on the lower back. The person with dementia may not be able to verbalize back pain or nerve tin-
gling or pain in the legs. Additionally, lying on the side and
turning from side to side allows the upside lung to completely
expand, aiding in prevention of pneumonia.

The side lying position can be enhanced by the use of pillows.
After being certain the person is **completely on his/her
side**, place a pillow in front of the body so the upper arm is
supported. Failure to place the person totally on his/her side
and propping with pillows in the partially turned position
creates more stress on the back than any other position in
bed. Additionally, it places most of the person's weight on the
back of the shoulder and the hip bone, contributing to the
formation of pressure sores. The complete side position promotes a relaxed posture, aiding the sleep process. Additionally, a pillow may be placed between the person's knees, if
desired. Alternatively, the down side leg can be partially
straightened with the upside leg bent and the upside knee
resting on the mattress. This position is referred to as the
"back neutral" position by back specialists.

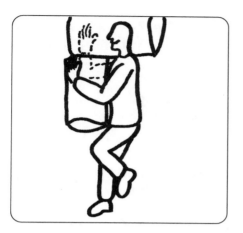

Back Neutral Position
Correct

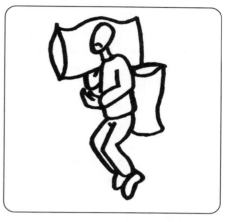

Side Lying Position
Incorrect

Tips for Getting into and out of an Automobile

It can be very difficult for persons with dementing illness to get in and out of a car seat with ease. With cognitive decline, logical and habitual steps for doing so are forgotten. I have observed persons with dementing illness in all kinds of contorted positions attempting to get into a car. Both safety and discomfort are issues. The following procedural steps will make this process easier both for the caregiver and the person with dementia.

- Park the car on a flat surface far enough from the curb so the person can step onto the street and turn to sit.

- Move the front seat back as far as possible to allow for ease of movement. The front seat is more easily accessible.

- If car seats are made of velour or cloth material, cover with a more slippery material, such as a sheet of plastic to make turning and shifting easier.

- With the front door open, maneuver the person around so that his/her buttocks are facing the side of the car seat (turn his/her back toward the car). Either hold the person's hands in yours, or place the left hand on the door and the right hand on the back of the front door frame. Back the person up until the back of his/her legs are touching the car seat.

- With feet remaining outside of the car and firmly on the ground, have the person sit sideways on the seat, appropriately cueing and/or guiding.

- After the person is seated, cue to put first the left leg, then the right leg into the car, swiveling around to face the front of the car. Make necessary adjustments such as scooting to the back of the seat.

- Buckle up!

8

MAINTAINING A SAFE AND COMFORTABLE ENVIRONMENT

What if you continually tripped over a scatter rug, or bumped into a table, or stumbled over a box on the floor, but couldn't determine how to correct the situation? What if you looked and felt like you were going to fall each time you were trying to pull up your pants, but did not have enough cognitive ability to determine the need to sit in a chair to start dressing?

Providing a safe environment is a major responsibility of the caregiver. As the person with dementia progresses in illness, the ability to perform many every day functions decreases. For example, whereas, the person formerly may have been able to stand to dress, balance decreases so that standing to dress becomes unsafe. In these situations, prevention of falls and complications from falls is a major role of the caregiver. An alert caregiver must constantly observe for actual and potential safety problems, and take corrective action to avoid accidents.

Corrective action may include, but is not limited to: removing unsafe objects or personal care items; rearranging furniture;

disconnecting cooking elements or microwave ovens; or retraining the person to perform some activities of daily living in a safe manner by changing written or verbal cues.

Maintaining body warmth is a frequent problem of the older adult. The person with dementia may not be able to verbalize being too cold or too hot. Early signs of the need for warmer room temperatures may be that the person wants to wear a coat inside, or wear clothing to bed. Therefore, it is important for the caregiver not only to question the person regarding being too warm or too cold, but in addition, to feel the person's hands and/or feet to see that they are appropriately warm. The older adult is usually much more comfortable in rooms with temperatures in the middle to upper 70s. The caregiver may have to dress in light clothing to be comfortable in this environment.

Layering of light clothing may be beneficial. However, layering of heavy and/or bulky clothing may inhibit upper body muscle movement, an undesirable situation for a person who needs to utilize as many muscles as possible to stay fit. Flannel sheets feel soft and cozy as well as providing additional warmth in winter and coolness in summer.

The person with dementing illness may be very sensitive to hot and cold water as well. Hot water heater thermostats should be turned down, so there is no chance the person can be burned accidentally. Lukewarm water may be preferred for drinking or oral hygiene.

The issue of smoking is a difficult one. Certainly safety is one problem. The person with dementia may leave burning cigarettes in inappropriate places or fall asleep with a cigarette in hand. If smoking is to be continued it must be done with supervision. However, the caregiver has to evaluate the overall effects of cigarette smoking, as well. Smoking contributes to the incidence of heart disease, lung disease, strokes, and hypertension. Additionally, smoking may have a direct effect on both the physical and intellectual functioning abilities of the person with dementia. The blood vessel constricting properties of nicotine decrease blood flow to the brain, which already is compromised from the diseases leading to the dementia condition.

Another difficult issue is that of when and how to stop the person with dementing illness from driving. Driving an automobile requires not only habitual skills, but also muscle coordination and cognitive functioning. **Persons with dementia do not have appropriate judgment to handle an automobile safely.** I have seen persons with dementia driving unsafely for months before something is done. Behaviors such as speeding, driving on the wrong side of the road, cutting across parking lots, and failure to stop for signs or lights are common with persons driving with dementia. Accidents frequently cause the person with dementia to panic and to flee the scene, thus adding hit-and-run driving to the problem. Certainly, defensive driving or ability to avoid an accident are not within the realm of the person with dementia. It may take every bit of brain power left just to keep the vehicle on the road and remember where he/she is going or how to get home.

Since driving becomes a major safety issue not only for the person with dementia, but also for others who may be harmed in an accident, the caregiver must pursue this problem expediently. Ride with the person to determine safety. Ask others who may have observed driving habits or ridden with the person if he/she is driving safely.

Several options may be available or functional in stopping the person with dementia from driving. The most loving and trust engendering approach is an honest one. Discuss the problems with the person with dementing illness. Tell him/her he/she is unsafe and cannot drive any longer. Do not come armed with a laundry list of all of his/her driving mistakes. This will only provide fuel for arguments. Make arrangements for other safe transportation so the person can get where he/she wants to go.

If the caregiver cannot bring him/herself to addressing this issue directly, contact the Department of Licensing in your state to determine available options. Many states will send a letter requiring the person to take a driver's examination. Some states will ask for a medical evaluation as a means of determining driving safety. Seeking assistance from a physician to tell the person with dementia he/she is no longer able to drive is another option available to caregivers. However, I strongly encourage loving family members telling the person honestly and directly.

9

MAINTAINING MUSCLE TONE AND GENERAL BODY CONDITIONING

The aging adult, and particularly a person with dementing illness, has increasing difficulties with maintaining physical fitness. Decrease in mental functioning may lead to social isolation, resulting in withdrawal from normal activities which require the utilization of muscles. Brain deterioration may lead to destruction of nerve pathways and processes which tell the muscles to function.

Another problem in older adults with poor muscle tone is that weight loss tends to result in loss of muscle. Therefore, any illness or accident requiring bed rest or inactivity, renders the person almost functionless physically. The person who has good muscle tone and endurance prior to illness or injury will recover much more quickly than the person without.

The person with dementing illness, if started on a specific exercise program in the early stages, can delay and/or slow the process of physical decline. Good muscle tone is essential for maintaining normal body functions such as evacuating bowel movements, and for maintainining posture and mobility. Additionally, good muscle tone will strengthen bones to prevent osteoporosis and will assist in maintaining body balance and movement, thereby preventing potential injury from falls.

There are three aspects of maintaining muscle tone that are important to the caregiver. One is that of utilizing all possible muscles while performing every day activities; the second is in encouraging muscle usage when the person is relaxing; and the third is initiation of a more formal exercise program.

Maintaining Muscle Tone in Performing Routine Activities

One of the most difficult processes for a caregiver is to stand by and watch a person with dementing illness trying to perform routine activities, such as getting out of a chair, sitting up in bed, or dressing. The extremely slowed thought processes, and sometimes, confusion, lead to a very slow response time. It becomes all too easy for the caregiver to assist the person by pulling, pushing, or doing. Nothing is more harmful for the person with dementia.

I would suggest as you are reading this section that you stop for a few minutes and practice doing some simple activities such as those discussed above—getting out of a chair or sitting up in bed. Do them slowly and deliberately and feel each of the muscles you utilize when performing the activity. Imagine what would happen if each of the muscles you detect you are using has become so weak that you could no longer perform the activity. If you, as a caregiver, assist the person with dementia in performing any movement, you will hasten muscle weakness, thereby fostering physical dependence on yourself or others.

Observed experiences with my father serve to emphasize the importance of physically independent functioning. At the time my father began showing symptoms of cognitive impairment, I was living 1,000 miles away and visited only about six times a year. By the time I had made the decision to move near my parents and participate in their caregiving, my very helpful mother had assisted my father in performing so many physical activities that he was not even able to get out of a chair without assistance. His leg, arm, and abdominal muscles had deteriorated markedly, making it very difficult to perform routine activities without assistance.

Three months subsequent to my relocation, after finally getting Mother to understand the problems her helpfulness was creating, Dad was once again able to get out of a chair by himself, and perform many of the other activities he had been unable to accomplish previously. I did initiate a formal program of planned, scheduled exercise for him which increased the speed of his muscle reconditioning.

Remember, it is extremely important that the person with dementing illness perform any and all activities independently, if possible. Even the slightest motions such as reaching, pushing, putting on jackets, getting out of bed, or up from a chair without assistance will contribute to improved muscle tone. Additionally, independent performance of activities will increase feelings of achievement and accomplishment and serve to enhance the quality of life for the person with dementing illness.

Encouraging Muscle Utilization When Relaxing

There are many times during the day when caregivers can encourage persons with dementing illness to strengthen muscles by being a little creative. When the person is listening to music, encourage arm movements, clapping hands, or tapping toes in time to the music. Encourage activities such as dancing, which promote good posture and utilize many muscle groups.

When walking by someone who is sitting in a chair, entice him/her to reach up and try to touch your hands, either one arm at a time, or both arms at once. Alternatively, say, "Suzy, how high can you reach today?" Raising both arms and reaching higher with first one arm and then the other is a great gentle stretching exercise. When walking by someone who is sitting in a chair, encourage the person to strengthen quadriceps muscles in the upper thigh by asking him/her to hold a leg out straight to a count of 5 or 10. This action will also stretch the backs of the leg. Encourage the person to hold his/her leg out straight and move the foot up and down. This is extremely relaxing, as well as strengthening in nature. Do only one leg at a time to protect the back from injury.

If you notice the person is sitting out of alignment, cue for appropriate alignment. If you see the person's head cocked to the side, encourage straightening the neck. Assist the person to get his/her head upright. The person may not know where straight up and down is. Suggest neck loosening exercises such as moving the head up and down and turning it side to side. If arms and legs are continually crossed or pulled inward, encourage outward stretching of arms and legs. Encourage sitting with feet at least shoulder width apart. All of these activities will make muscles tired from inactivity feel better, as well as prevent muscle and tendon tightening and contracting.

Developing and Maintaining Muscle Mass Through a Program of Planned Exercise

There is a growing amount of research which shows the benefit of planned exercise for the aging adult. A major role of the care-giver is to see that planned exercise is included and executed in a daily schedule. **No exercise program should be initiated without the approval and consent of a physician.**

Major objectives in planning exercise for the aging adult and the person with dementing illness are: to increase muscle tone to improve physical functioning; to increase flexibility and balance; to improve physical stamina or endurance; and to reduce stress and promote a feeling of well-being.

Planned exercise minimally should include the following:

*   Aerobic activity—at least 3 times a week for 20 minutes, spaced throughout the week.

    If the person with dementia cannot tolerate 20 minutes of continual movement, recent research is showing that exercise can be broken into shorter blocks which total 20 to 30 minutes for the day.

    Usually walking, even slow walking, is aerobic for many aging adults. Calculation of the heart rate necessary to maintain an aerobic state is different for the aging adult. As age increases, the heart rate needed to perform aerobically decreases. **Generally, a 10 second pulse rate between 15**

and 19 will be more than adequate to sustain aerobic functioning in an adult between the ages of 70 and 90.

More indepth information on aerobic exercise and the need to perform warm up and stretching exercises before and after is included in Appendix E3. Please refer to this section before doing aerobic activity.

◆ Exercises designed to promote flexibility, range of motion, and balance—daily.

Depth and spatial perceptual difficulties are prevalent in persons with dementia. Aerobic exercise will promote cardiac and respiratory fitness, but will not promote balance or flexibility and range of motion of all joints. Working with flexibility and range of motion of all body muscles and joints is crucial to maintaining the person with dementia in an ambulatory state.

The old saying, "use it or lose it," really pertains here. Without stretching and utilizing all muscles, some will become stretched and others contracted, resulting in inability to utilize some muscles altogether. Typically, problems occur in the shoulders, arms, and legs. The more a person sits, the more permanently bent he/she will become, until, persons sitting constantly in a chair will become almost "chair shaped," and will not be able to straighten their hips, arms, or legs. How sad it is to see this happening to those with dementing illness, when daily stretching and movement of all muscles would prevent the problem entirely. Caregivers must realize how **extremely painful** it is when muscles become weak, contracted, and out of alignment from lack of use. Have you ever been in one position too long, and hurt when you began to move? Imagine being in one position constantly, e.g., sitting in a chair.

Detailed, safe exercises for warm up and range of motion are included in Appendix E2. Please refer to this section before doing any form of exercise.

◆ Exercises designed to tone all body muscles, including work with **light weights**—three times per week.

Aerobic activities and range of motion and balance exercises generally will not maintain or improve muscle strength. Recent research with older persons in nursing homes demonstrates remarkable improvement in physical functioning of those on a muscle toning program. I am not suggesting a major body building program, just working with light weights.

At the beginning stages of weight exercises, it is best to perform the motions without weights for at least two weeks. Gradually add weights at monthly intervals starting with one pound (or $\frac{1}{2}$ pound) and increase as tolerated up to a maximum of three pounds. Most older women can improve muscle performance with continuous work with one pound weights. Men may require more. The numbers of repetitions should be no more than eight to ten. With any complaints of pain, muscle tenderness, or soreness, weight activities should be stopped.

Specific toning exercises are detailed in Appendix E4. Please refer to that section before doing any toning exercises.

Specific exercises for each of the above categories are included in Appendix E of this book. **Please check with a physician before embarking on any exercise program.**

Utilizing Exercise Equipment

Exercise bicycles can be utilized with ease by many people with dementing illness. This activity is especially good for those who may have ridden bicycles when they were younger. Long periods of cycling may not be tolerated. However, even short rides are beneficial, not only for cardiovascular conditioning, but also for strengthening the front leg muscles and lengthening the muscles in the backs of the legs. The seat must be adjusted so that when the pedal is at the bottom of the loop, the leg is fully extended—nearly straight. Otherwise, the back leg muscles will not be stretched. Cycling to music may be very relaxing, as well as extremely beneficial from an exercise standpoint.

Stair climbers may be a little too vigorous in nature for cardio-vascular conditioning for the older adult. However, stair climbers can be very beneficial for strengthening the leg, lower back, and buttocks muscles, and for stretching the backs of the legs. For persons doing a lot of sitting who are beginning to have difficulty straightening their legs, utilization of a stair climber for very brief periods will be of great value. For safety reasons, only stair climbers with grab bars should be utilized. However, it is important to **cue for upright posture rather than forward leaning posture** when doing stair climber work.

Treadmills also may be too vigorous for most older people to utilize for cardiovascular conditioning. However, if used even for brief periods, there will be benefits as a leg muscle strengthening mechanism. Treadmills with firm grab bars can be very beneficial for the person having problems with balance, who otherwise may not be able to walk for any distance. Manual treadmills are preferable to motorized treadmills, as the person with dementing illness can control the speed completely. Motorized treadmills not only may be unsafe, but also can be very frightening to a person with dementing illness who may not be able to express his/her need to either slow down or stop the treadmilling activity.

The newest piece of exercise equipment which may be extremely beneficial and safe for those with dementing illness is the gravity rider—several brands are available. These machines have bicycle-like seats, with handle bars and foot pedals. The person holds onto the handle bars and pulls him/herself to a standing position. Designed for effective cardiovascular conditioning, muscle toning, and muscle stretching, these machines are wonderful and can frequently be utilized by the person with dementia with minimal supervision. Because the seat is low to the floor, it is easy for the caregiver to assist in positioning the person on the seat. Mother loved to get on a gravity rider and pull herself to a standing position. This workout greatly relieved muscle tension in nearly all areas of her body. Again, most people with dementia cannot endure long workouts on cardiovascular equipment, but just a few minutes at a slow place makes the person feel great! Just be certain that the machine is durable, and does not have a tendency to tip. The more expensive machines will be safe to use.

Again, to prevent injury, I stress the importance of doing appropriate warm up exercises before exercising, including using exercise equipment. Additionally, stretching exercises must be done following the use of any exercise equipment. Refer to Appendix E for appropriate warm up and stretching exercises.

The Use of Exercise Cue Cards

Exercise cue cards can be an excellent tool for allowing the person with dementing illness to exercise at his/her own pace, while at the same time, providing mental stimulation from reading and following a set exercise sequence. Once individual exercises are learned, and specific names or cues are attached, they can be placed on large index cards. Using colored marking pens, cards can be numbered sequentially. Develop cues of only 3-4 words so they may be easily read and understood. Mother was able to do her routines for years without verbal coaching. She took great pride in methodically reading each cue card, performing the exercise, and turning the card upside down to indicate she had completed that exercise. I made her cue cards in huge print in dark black letters because of her diminished vision due to macular degeneration.

10

PROMOTING MENTAL AND INTELLECTUAL FUNCTIONING

Promoting the highest level of mental and intellectual functioning is a primary challenge for the caregiver. Caregiver frustration can occur when having to continually cue and re-cue the person with dementia to encourage independent functioning. It is all too easy to give up in exasperation and actually perform the function for the person with dementing illness. I can only encourage caregivers to do all in their power to maintain patience and provide the time for the slow and painstaking process of cueing the person with dementing illness to perform activities for him/herself. The rewards for the caregiver and the obvious self-satisfaction of the person with dementia far outweigh any frustration suffered in the process.

It is essential to know the mental capabilities of the person with dementia prior to determining processes and activities that will be utilized to enhance these capabilities. It is particularly important to know the person's ability to read and to understand, and ability to follow verbal instructions. The person who cannot follow written instructions is not a candidate for written cueing.

Assuming the person can do both, the following methods will encourage active brain activity:

- At the beginning of every day orient the person as to the day of the week, the date and the year. Loss of the concept of time is prevalent in the person with dementia. For the person in early stages, the caregiver might ask the person if he/she knows what the date, year, and day are? Also orient to up-coming holidays, and other special events. Reinforce this time and place orientation as necessary throughout the day. Utilizing a calendar and having the person with dementia cross off the days as they occur can be effective.

- At the beginning of every day and more frequently, if necessary, discuss activities for the day, so the person with dementia will know what is coming next. If reviewing the entire day's events is too complicated, just let the person know what the next activity will be. Provide a written schedule for the day, posted in a specific place to be viewed throughout the day as necessary.

- Review major world and local events at a set time each day, either by having the person read the headlines, or by the caregiver reading and discussing news events with the person with dementia. Slow and deliberate discussion is much more effective than turning on television news which is spoken too quickly and in sentences too long for a person with dementia to understand.

- If tasks such as dressing and other activities of personal care are too complicated for the person to remember the entire sequence, break them down into small groups of tasks that are more easily cued and more readily remembered.

- Make every attempt to maintain the lifestyle the person followed in the past. To the extent that old habits and practices can be continued, skills requiring cognitive functioning will decline more slowly. Familiar activities and familiar timing of activities make it easier for the person with dementing illness to remember and be functional.

- Maintain contacts with friends and relatives. Encourage conversation (utilizing communication techniques outlined earlier) about familiar people, places, and things. One of the most difficult aspects of progressive dementia is the loss of contact with familiar people. Frequently the person moves from the area. Even if the person stays in familiar surroundings, people close to the person are uncomfortable and don't know what to say. The caregiver can assist the person with dementia in communicating with friends and relatives through verbal cueing and suggesting contacts, such as writing cards, making phone calls, etc. Assisting the person to send birthday or other greeting cards and gifts is especially helpful, because this action promotes the return of gifts and cards from friends and relatives.

- Verbally cue the person to assist the memory function. Ask leading questions to which the person may know answers and that will trigger memory tie-ins to answers the person may not know. For example, if the caregiver is asking the question "What month is this?" and the person cannot respond, (and the month is December, for example), ask the question, "In which month is the Christmas holiday?" This same approach can be utilized in triggering persons to remember names, events, etc. Then praise the person for the correct response.

* Encourage mentally stimulating as well as **functional** activities. For example, sorting mismatched socks, walking the dog, cleaning out a tool box, making the bed, and performing other activities of daily living, housekeeping, or maintenance tasks will give the person a sense of accomplishment and foster thought processes. The caregiver may want to plan simple projects in which the person with dementia can assist. The major objective is not to keep the person busy or happy, but rather to keep the person functional and more important, **feeling that he/she is functional. Even if the job is only half completed or done poorly, the person will still feel useful and needed.**

* Incorporate actual mental exercises such as counting, doing math problems, writing, reciting the alphabet, spelling, singing old songs or reciting nursery rhymes into daily activities. Encourage playing checkers or bingo or scrabble if the person is cognitively capable. Counting money in a wallet or billfold can be mentally stimulating as well as useful in nature.

* Encourage activities that were typical activities prior to developing dementia. For example, if watching the financial channel or following stocks in the newspaper or watching specific television programs were daily activities prior to the onset of dementing illness, provide time in the schedule and caregiver assistance and encouragement to enable the person to continue to perform these activities.

* Plan for and encourage activities that are just plain recreational for a break from the more functional, mind stimulating activities. Persons with dementia who have had to give up driving and movement independence may enjoy getting out for automobile rides. Encourage continuing participation

in activities such as golf, pool, bowling, baseball, swimming, and social clubs.

◆   Utilizing some type of music for recreational activities can be extremely beneficial for persons with dementia. Frequently, hearing popular music from earlier years will prompt the person with dementing illness to begin singing or dancing. Music is very relaxing. Remembering words to older songs is mind stimulating. Dancing is wonderful exercise. Mother had a great deal of rhythm far into the disease process. We frequently danced. Due to her stroke, I had to do a lot of supporting, but it was worth the extra effort just to see her kick up her heels, so to speak.

◆   Plan for participation in **small** group activities, if possible, to prevent social isolation. Persons with dementia cannot manage large numbers of contacts or contact with people that they have not seen for a long time. As the dementia causing disease progresses, even frequently seen relatives and friends may not be recognized. Placing a person with dementia in a situation where he/she is expected to socialize or remember many people is very stressful. Keep groups to the smallest size possible. Groups of two or three very familiar people may be the most the person with dementia can manage. It is better to invite friends into your loved one's environment than to take your loved one to a strange setting.

◆   Encourage social communication skills with others. For example, upon meeting someone say, "Oh, there's (Suzy), let's go say hello to her." Or, if someone speaks to the person with dementia and there is no response, say "Mother (or name of person), did you hear (Suzy) say hello?" or whatever the appropriate question and response should be.

- Celebrate holidays and special occasions with small groups and lots of decorating to create a festive type of mood. Older people in general, and especially those with dementing illnesses respond to happy times with bright colors. Utilizing items such as balloons, party hats, and bright bouquets are just a few suggestions for bringing happiness and responsiveness to the person with dementia.

Some activities that may not work for persons with dementing illness are reading, playing cards, watching television, or going to a movie. It is important to remember that each of these activities requires a great deal of cognitive ability. If one can't remember the beginning of a sentence before getting to the end, one certainly can't remember how to play cards or follow the story line of a movie or a book or follow the news report in depth. However, watching a musical event on television, or attending a musical production or movie may be very relaxing, providing a group situation such as a theater is not anxiety producing. Mother enjoyed watching Lawrence Welk program repeats and figure skating on television.

Sharing an experience I had week after week with Mother will underscore the importance of mind stimulating activities. She was in a skilled nursing facility part time, and with me part time in the last few years. During her last year of life, when I arrived at the nursing facility to take her home with me, she either was not able to tell me who she was, and/or was unable to identify me by name. After spending a great deal of time in talking with her and being certain she was comfortable in getting in the car and going home with me, we would leave the building. As we exited the parking lot, I encouraged her to sing her college fight song, knowing she never forgot the words to that song. Following singing the song, I asked Mother to tell me her name. Invariably, she could tell me her first name, and sometimes her last name. Next we would recite a nursery rhyme or two. I would start off with the beginning of a rhyme and she would fill in the remainder. After each successful recitation of a rhyme or song, I would ask her another question regarding her name, my name, and other family member names. By the time we arrived at my home 30 minutes later, she always knew her name, my name, and my father's and brother's names.

Mother always told me, when she had regained her sense of self, that she knew from the beginning, but was not able to express the names. She also told me she was much more relaxed and comfortable after regaining her ability to express that which she had been unable to do previously. Just as demonstrated during the cueing process discussed in Chapter 6, Mother was visibly more relaxed and conversational when she was assisted with her memory by singing familiar songs or reciting familiar nursery rhymes.

It is amazing what will occur when you work with the person with dementia to stimulate and encourage mental activities. Most people are extremely surprised at how much thought capacity the person with dementing illness has. Unfortunately, frequently these thought processes are not cultivated deeply enough to reap the benefit of these experienced and wise minds. I encourage you to make every attempt to elicit input from persons with dementing illness. The person's life will be more meaningful, and your life will be enriched in so doing.

11

THE IMPORTANCE OF STRUCTURING AND SCHEDULING

It is important that caregivers provide as much structure as is possible for the person with dementing illness. Structure means having events scheduled at the same time every day. This allows the person with dementia to learn the pattern, and begin to know what is coming next. Activities such as meal times, bathing, oral hygiene, sleeping and resting, private time, exercising, letter writing, telephoning, newspaper reading, TV watching, and all other repetitive activities must be scheduled in writing. The more activities are repetitive in both content and time, the more control the person with dementia feels he/she has. Control promotes a feeling of accomplishment and self-confidence. Schedules and structure create a greater sense of predictability and security for the person with dementia.

A schedule of routines and activities cannot be determined arbitrarily. The person with dementing illness should be involved as much as is possible in the planning process. Utilize the schedule as a prompting tool. When questioned by the person with dementia as to "What is happening next?," refer him/her to this schedule. This assumes, of course, there are no vision or reading comprehension problems. Post it in a place where it can be found easily. Use big bold writing. Utilize pictures and bright colors to make it colorful, interesting, and informative. If vision is a problem, frequent discussion of the schedule is extremely important so the person with dementing illness can become familiar with daily events.

Providing enough time for each activity is of particular importance. The older person, and particularly one with dementia, may be painstakingly slow in performing any activity, whether intellectual or physical. It is crucial for the caregiver to stand back and patiently observe as the person with dementing illness performs tasks, offering cueing only if absolutely necessary. The old saying, "patience is a virtue," is extremely applicable in caregiving for persons with dementing illness.

Additionally, once a schedule is determined, it should not be cast in concrete. It is important to evaluate and revise the schedule to meet the needs and changing conditions of the person with dementing illness.

Occasional deviation from the schedule for unplanned events that are of particular interest to the person with dementia is appropriate and recommended.

Some persons with dementia cannot handle rigid scheduling of activities. However, many who seem agitated and are wandering are really searching for assistance and will respond to more environmental structure and control. You, as caregiver, will have to evaluate your individual situation. One of the most complex and perplexing problems in working with people with dementia, is that each person is different in his/her response to the environment. Not only does each individual respond differently, but also the same person may respond differently from hour to hour, day to day, or month to month. These changes in response really challenge the caregiver to be creative and patient in providing the correct amount of environmental structure and control to maintain a balance between keeping the person with dementing illness more functional and promoting a feeling of having intellectual independence.

12

PREVENTING UNNECESSARY ANXIETY AND STRESS

Philosophical Position

I believe the primary caregiver has a major responsibility for preventing unnecessary anxiety and stress in the person with dementing illness. I believe therapeutic caregiving, administered appropriately, will both predict and prevent many anxiety producing situations. Further, I believe that many so-called *"catastrophic events,"* or behavior outbursts, can be prevented by keeping stressful situations to a minimum.

Why Prevent Stress?

There long has been an understanding of the ill effects of high stress levels on our bodies. Stress contributes to physical conditions such as high blood pressure, stomach problems and heart attacks. Stress contributes to psychological and emotional problems, as well. The person with dementing illness is no different from the rest of us in terms of the physiological and psychological effects of stress.

However, due to the difficulties in adapting to and coping with stressful situations, stress effects are magnified in the person with dementia. Two things seem to happen to persons with dementia when they are in a stressed state. The first is a reduced ability to function at all levels. The stress producing problem seems to consume their entire being. The second may be a severe reaction frequently referred to as a *"catastrophic event."* Reactions such as refusing to eat, total withdrawal, spitting, accusing their loved ones of being against them, throwing things, hitting, biting, kicking, among others, are classified as catastrophic events. I don't like the use of the term "catastrophic," because I think of a catastrophic event as being uncontrollable. A lot of so-called agressive behavior is actually protective, defensive, or reactive in nature—reactive to perceived threats or overwhelming anxiety. I strongly believe many of these events can be minimized, if not controlled by a knowledgeable and perceptive caregiver.

It is very difficult for those of us with normal cognitive capacities to imagine how frightening it must feel to literally be losing your sense of mind and of self. Have you ever lost your wallet or your purse, or misplaced your car keys? Have you ever been in a very anxiety producing situation such as an auto accident? Can you identify any situation in which you were very frightened and felt out of control? Do you recall how you could not focus on anything else and how overwhelmed you felt? I am asking these questions only to stimulate you as a reader of this book to recall how you felt in a very stressful situation.

Now recall some of the "what if" questions posed and situations presented in previous chapters. What if you couldn't remember important people, places, and events? What if you needed to urinate, but couldn't express your needs? What if you couldn't remember how to get into your bathroom? How would you feel if you were in a family gathering and were so overwhelmed you couldn't remember the names of those closest to you? Much of the information presented in previous chapters will give you insight into the kinds of situations that can be anxiety producing for the person with dementing illness.

Behaviors Indicative of Anxiety

If you can recall the way you felt in stressful times and during anxious moments, you will remember some of the behaviors you displayed. Sleeplessness, pacing, inability to focus, crying, angry outbursts, and withdrawal, may be some of the behaviors you exhibited. These behaviors are no different from those you may see in someone with dementing illness. There may be major differences in the events or situations that trigger anxiety, however, due to the greatly diminished cognitive capacity of the person with dementia. As a caregiver, you need to be aware not only of the obvious signs of anxiety, but also of the subtle questions or behaviors that may indicate your loved one is in a stressful situation.

Following is a brief listing of some of the subtle examples (comments, questions, observations) I have noticed which are indicative of anxiety or potential anxiety producing events.

• "The cars are going so fast."

- "That car is passing on the right."

- "I'm glad I'm not driving any more."

- "I can't remember Suzy's phone number."

- "I can't find my keys."

- "These trees are so tall."

- "How many people will be there?"

- "Where are we?"

- A blank look when asked a question.

- Sitting and looking down when communicating, rather than using eye contact.

- Somewhat frantic rocking in a rocking chair.

- Difficulty in swallowing.

- Talking with a strained voice.

This brief and certainly incomplete list serves to indicate some of the key stress producing problems for persons with dementia.

One problem is that of difficulty with actual perception of such things as speed, heights, distances, etc. Therefore, feeling like the car is going too fast or fearing what may happen with tall trees are frequently heard comments. I have heard them from all three people with whom I have been more intimately involved in caregiving. The comment about someone passing on

the right tells the caregiver the person with dementia is thinking back to the days when roads were one lane in each direction.
The only correct way to pass was on the left. Reassurance in all
these instances will allow the person to relax and feel safe in the
hands of a trusted caregiver. As an example one might say, "You
are thinking about passing on the left." "Is that correct?" After
waiting for a response you might say, "Roads have several lanes
now." "It is permissible to pass on the right." "Remember the
days when roads weren't so crowded?" Hopefully this last question will promote discussion of earlier times, something people
with dementing illness can do well into the disease process.
Discussion of earlier times may be a good distraction from the
condition that is causing stress.

A second problem is one discussed earlier in this book. I am
repeating it to lend emphasis. Persons with dementing illness
simply cannot function in large groups. There is too much stimulation coming at once, and a total inability to process what is
happening. As the disease progresses, groups will become more
and more anxiety producing to the point that your loved one will
literally not be able to function. It may make some difference in
earlier stages if a trusted caregiver is close at hand and can
assist the person in responding and adapting. Structured and
low-stimulation environments may help initially. However, as
the dementia process progresses, exposure to large groups may
cause an obvious anxiety reaction, such as inability to eat or
swallow, bolting out of a room, an outburst of anger, wanting to
go home, or total withdrawal, among others. As dementia progresses, groups of three may seem large, and in some instances,
relating to one trusted person is all that is tolerated. If you, as a
caregiver, find that the person for whom you are caregiving is
showing signs of anxiety or decrease in functional ability, excuse
yourselves and get into a more familiar environment or into a

more private place, even if it means leaving someone's home or exiting from the scene as a host or hostess.

A third problem creating stress in the person with dementing illness is that of being incapable of performing simple sequential tasks. The comment about not remembering someone's phone number may be much more complex than what is at the surface. It is much easier to say you have forgotten someone's phone number than it is to admit that you can't dial a complete phone number or don't remember how to use the phone. Caregivers frequently ask the person with dementia to contact them if they need something. For example, "Call me when you need to go to the bathroom," sounds like a reasonable request. "Telephone me when you need more groceries," is another similar request. However, these requests are impossible for the person with dementia to execute. They require recall of recent events or use of short term memory, the very portion of memory that leaves first in the dementia process.

Utilizing the telephone may become impossible early in the dementia process. The person with dementing illness may be able to talk via telephone even into advanced stages of the disease. However, dialing a telephone number or using a memory phone may be impossible. Mother was able to do it for quite a while because I set up her memory phone very early on, and use of the memory buttons had become more habitual to her.

However, dialing a 10 digit number is impossible. Even if the number is written in large print, the person with dementia will forget what number has just been dialed before getting to the end of the telephone number. Typically, the first two or three digits will go fine, but the remainder will be lost and become a source of major frustration and stress. Memory phones requiring pushing only one or two buttons can work fairly well if the process is learned in early stages of the dementia process. If your phone requires you to push a memory function key, you may have to color it in red and train the person to push the red button and then the appropriate number to initiate automatic dialing of the telephone number.

A fourth stress creating problem is that of losing items of importance. We all misplace items occasionally, but I am certain you can recall a time when you temporarily lost something of great importance and remember how stressed you were. It is not uncommon for someone with dementing illness to continually lose items of importance—keys, dentures, jewelry, watches, and purses or wallets are frequently misplaced. Since recent recall and short term memory are lost, the difficulty in locating objects is sabotaged on several fronts. The person not only may not remember where he/she left the object of importance, but also may not remember exactly what it looks like. Those of us who have normal cognitive capacities would have the capacity to find the missing object, assuming it was just misplaced. However, the person with dementia usually will not be able to find misplaced items. It is not unusual to find the person fixating on looking for the object, even to the point of neglecting to sleep or eat until it is found. I used to telephone one person with dementing illness daily in the early morning, because I knew he would not be able to find something, such as his house key, and would not be able to function, including eating breakfast, until he did. I could usually tell him where he might look to find the key. I would stay on the line until he came back to the phone and said he had found the key.

One way to reduce the possibility of misplacing important items is to have specific places labeled for important and frequently utilized items. For example, there would be a dish or box labeled for a watch, another for a ring, another for a wallet, keys, etc. The daughter of my friend with dementia assisted her father to find his keys by placing a huge fluorescent orange plasticized tag on the key ring. It is important to start conditioning the person with dementing illness to have a set spot for important items early on in the dementia process.

A fifth problem is that of not knowing where he/she is. Have you ever been lost with no one to assist you? The person with dementia may become lost in a neighborhood, or within his/her own home. It is not in the least uncommon to find that a person with dementing illness becomes lost while driving. What a frightening feeling this must be. My friend, Bruce, before he was getting appropriate assistance, left his residence in a retirement community in the middle of the night. Several of the buildings looked similar in his complex. For some reason he had a key that fit another residence which had an entrance that looked exactly like his. He went in, used the rest room, and left his coffee cup on the dining room table before he left—all while the residence owners were fast asleep. It must have been a terrifying feeling to think he was in his own residence and find nothing that was familiar. Needless to say, the people whose residence was entered were not thrilled, either.

I could go on and on with examples of potential stress producing situations. However, my point is not to present a laundry list of stress producing situations, but rather to emphasize the constant state of turmoil your loved one may be experiencing in just trying to hold on to a sense of self and carry out normal activities of daily living.

If anyone is reading this book out of concern for someone with memory problems and that person is living alone, I implore you to do everything in your power to see that the living situation is changed so that the person with dementing illness has appropriate assistance essential to his/her functioning without undue stress and anxiety.

Preventing and Minimizing Stress

It is obvious that utilizing some of the techniques presented throughout this book, and particularly in this chapter, will be helpful in preventing stressful situations. Additionally, many activities that may be relaxing to the person with dementing illness will be helpful in preventing stress. Utilization of hobbies, music, walking, dancing, and art are only a few of the relaxing activities which come to mind. New fields in music and art therapy are emerging as the value of creative and relaxing activities is increasingly recognized.

People with dementing illness, and older people in general, respond wonderfully to cuddly pets. Mother loved to watch the birds and squirrels when she visited my home. I set up outdoor feeding stations a short distance away from a table perfect for enjoying meals or a cup of tea and watching the wildlife. Some friends of mine purchased a black and white bunny for Mother, after I told them how much Mother had enjoyed holding a bunny from the feed store one day when I was purchasing bird feed.

Cuddly stuffed animals may be appreciated and relaxing, as well. Mother loved little bears. She liked to talk with them, even though they didn't respond. One day I asked her what she liked about talking to her little bears. She told me, "She wasn't pressured to respond. She could say whatever she wanted." She especially liked a little bear who says "I love you," when you squeeze her little rump.

Physical exercise is essential to both preventing and reducing stress levels. It would be ideal if relaxing and fun activities such as walking or dancing could be incorporated into a schedule of planned daily exercise.

It goes without saying that if the caregiver is stressed, the person with dementing illness will be more stressed. Previously I indicated that it has been my experience and that of many caregivers that the person with dementia is even more sensitive to feelings and tones of voice than are those of us who are not cognitively impaired. When we are stressed we just plain have a "shorter fuse." We may anger more quickly, or may not be as keen on observing and resolving problems. As a caregiver, you must get respite, utilize relaxation techniques, and regularly participate in physical exercise sessions to promote a state of physical and emotional well-being in yourself. This state will be sensed and responded to by the person with dementing illness for whom you are the primary caregiver.

13

MANAGING PROBLEM BEHAVIORS

Are Terrible Behaviors Expected?

The general public is infused with the idea that if someone has a dementing illness such as Alzheimer's disease, terrible behavior problems can be **expected.** Many people picture someone with Alzheimer's disease as being agitated, aggressive, paranoid, and impossible to control. Family members are fearful that their loved ones with dementing illness will eventually turn into this awful person who is out of control, knows nothing and no one, and may harm him/her self or others. I believe people with dementing illness have acquired a stereotyped reputation which is not deserved.

My mother never displayed any aggressive or out of control behaviors. My father was very docile and easy to care for. It is entirely probable that your loved one will not have behavior problems. Maybe I was just lucky, but I would like to think that my actions and methods of relating to them helped avoid problem behaviors. I would caution caregivers that if you are conditioned to believing your loved one will have behavior problems, you will respond differently at the slightest sign of a problem, such as anger, for example. As part of therapeutic caregiving you need to take a look at yourself and how you respond to situations. Your response to your loved one's behavior can greatly influence the outcome.

I am not suggesting that problem behaviors do not occur with persons with dementing illness. Rather, I believe many of the aggressive and difficult behaviors about which we are accustomed to hearing are a result of caregivers not knowing how to recognize early signs of problems, not knowing how to analyze behaviors to determine the cause, and not knowing how to intervene when problem behaviors occur.

I fully recognize, however, that some behavior problems are caused by the disease process itself. These behaviors can be extremely upsetting to loved ones of those with dementing illness. I do not wish to diminish the difficulties and heartaches these behaviors cause. I have chosen not to address management of specific problem behaviors because other books, which are listed in the Complementary Reading Section in Appendix A, address specific behavior problems in great detail. Instead I will present appropriate concepts related to behavior, intervention techniques if a problem behavior occurs, and a method for analyzing problem behavior cycles as a method of prevention.

General Behavior Beliefs and Concepts

I believe that behavior in human beings is purposeful—that is we do what we do to meet some need. I further believe this purposeful behavior concept applies to persons with dementing illness as well as to the rest of us. I present these beliefs not as an educated psychologist, psychiatrist, or social worker, but as an observer of human behavior for more than 50 years. My rationale for presenting these beliefs is that if one believes behavior is purposeful, then it stands to reason that therapeutic caregiving would necessitate pulling back and taking a look at a particular behavior in terms of cause and effect.

Caregivers have been encouraged by many professionals to accept problem behaviors as part of the dementing disease process. This approach, in effect, totally avoids taking a look at the behavior, and trying to determine the cause and a potential solution to prevent repeats of the problem behavior. Both the caregiver and the person with dementia are losers in this situation. The caregiver endures a problem behavior, and the person with dementing illness may not be having his/her need(s) met. I strongly encourage a more analytical approach as the first line of attack, rather than assuming the disease is causing the problem behavior.

I think it is important for the therapeutic caregiver to realize that the person with dementing illness may have lost many of the social graces and inhibitions that have been in place throughout life. When those of us without cognitive deficits anger, most of us are a little careful in how we present ourselves in this anger stimulating situation. Most of us have learned appropriate manners and social standards for relating to others. The ability to think through appropriate social responses may have been lost in the person with dementing illness. Therefore, uninhibited responses occur. Caregivers need to understand this loss in cognitive ability if they wish to therapeutically intervene during an inappropriate display of behavior.

What to Do When a Problem Behavior Occurs

Many professionals recommend that caregivers make no attempt to intervene when a person with dementing illness is displaying a problem behavior unless there is potential for either self-harm or caregiver harm. These professionals are of the belief that problem behaviors are caused by the disease, and are, therefore, uncontrollable. Indeed, there may be no way to correct problem behaviors in some persons with dementia. However, if there is any possibility of changing the circumstances which cause the problem behavior, I believe both the person with dementia and the caregiver will benefit.

Caregivers must be aware of two primary considerations when managing problem behaviors. First and foremost, if the person for whom you are providing care is agitated and uncontrollable and may harm either him/herself or you, take whatever action is necessary from a safety standpoint. Persons with dementing illness, or any of the rest of us for that matter, in a severe state of agitation or anger can harm themselves or others. They physically can become very strong. Any attempt to be logical and rational may not work. Take action to protect yourself, the person, or others. Sometimes setting limits by saying something such as "I know you are very angry," (pause) "but I will not tolerate you hitting me," for example, may stop the behavior.

The second consideration is that of understanding that the way in which you, as a therapeutic caregiver, respond to the problem behavior will affect the behavior outcome. This concept is true in all human interaction situations, including those with persons with dementing illness. My own experience and that of many others with whom I have discussed this subject is that if the caregiver becomes upset or out of control, the problem behavior escalates. The more the behavior escalates, the more stressed the person with dementia becomes, leading to a decreasing level of cognitive functioning, and a decreasing ability to respond to a therapeutic approach.

It is extremely important for the caregiver to remain calm and objective in response to behavior problems. Remaining calm is particularly important when dealing with hostility or anger. I realize this is more easily said than done. It is particularly difficult to step out of a feeling, relational role into a therapeutic role if the caregiver perceives him/herself as a target of the behavior. I would encourage caregivers to step back from the situation, count to ten, or do whatever works to remove the emotional tones. Then step back in and attempt to intervene in a more objective but loving way. Process feelings with others—support groups, clergy, counselors, etc., to enable objectivity in the caregiving situation.

Remain calm and talk in soft and gentle tones with the person displaying the difficult behavior. Remember the tips on communication. Use gentle touching to reassure and calm the person. Use firm touching if you need to escort the person with dementing illness from the scene. Communicate caring and understanding both in tone of voice and in touch. Remember, the person displaying anger or agitation may be attempting to communicate something of importance about which he/she is very upset. This type of behavior may be the only way in which the person with dementia feels he/she can communicate.

One method of changing inappropriate behaviors is to try diversionary tactics. Attempt to get the person to move on to another subject. Remove the person from the environment in which the behavior is occurring, if this is appropriate. Suggesting it is time for a glass of juice, a snack, or to listen to music may be enough to change the focus from an undesirable behavior to a more acceptable activity.

Another technique the caregiver can use for minor and usually more impolite behavior problems or omissions is to cue or coach the person with dementing illness in such a way that the appropriate response occurs. There have been many instances in which I provided the socially acceptable cognitive processes in Mother's situation. She readily accepted coaching along this line, and never resisted my loving attempts to correct minor behavior problems or omissions that might have been offensive to others who didn't understand the dementing illness process. For example, when we were invited to a relative's home for a meal, Mother did not remember to thank the host/hostess for a nice evening. It was very easy for me to say something like, "Mother, it is time for us to leave." "Shall we thank (name) for the nice dinner." Mother then responded with appropriate salutations. This type of coaching action may seem totally unnecessary, but it accomplishes more than encouraging socially acceptable behavior. My actions assisted Mother to act in such a way that others had no choice but to respond to her. Everyone feels good in this type of interaction.

I also encourage gentle correcting of behavior that is not tolerated socially. Behaviors such as making sexual advances or fondling the genital area in a public place sometimes can be stopped with a gentle reminder. Other times the caregiver may have to escort the person from the scene and attempt to find a substitute activity to occupy his/her time and/or mind.

This may be an appropriate spot in which to mention the need for privacy and some time alone. No human being functions well with continual bombardment from other human beings. Quiet time away from people and other forms of mental stimulation is necessary to maintain a sense of self. Quiet time should be scheduled into daily activities. This is not to suggest that the person be left entirely alone and in an unsafe environment, rather that the caregiver retreat to another room or area while keeping a watchful eye and alert ears to be available to assist the person with dementing illness if necessary.

Previously I have discussed cueing for memory stimulation and assisting with logical thinking. This process necessitates the caregiver going back in time to the place where the person with dementing illness seems to be and working from there. A similar concept can be utilized in working with problem behaviors. Essentially, rather than attempting to stop the behavior by persuasion or by diversion to another activity, acknowledge the behavior and build on the responses. If the person is pacing or wandering, pace or wander with him/her. Get into the same rhythm and timing as the person with dementing illness. If the person is communicating a concern, pick up on the concern and talk about it. The following example may be of some assistance in understanding this technique.

The following event occurred one weekend, when I went to the skilled nursing facility where Mother resided, to take her home for the weekend. As I was passing through the corridor in the entry way, one of the residents was sitting in her wheel chair, arms stretched across a decorative table containing a floral arrangement, reaching and straining to hold onto the hand rail which spans the corridor. Her teeth were clenched and her grip on the rails so tight that her knuckles were white. She was obviously distressed about something. I approached her and asked, "Are you stuck?" She responded with, "No, they are robbing the place." I could have left the scene at that point, but decided to see if I could be of some assistance.

In working with persons with dementing illness I have found that behaviors and discussions frequently emanate from a past experience. So, I began to probe into the subject she presented. "What place are they robbing?" I asked. She responded with, "I am a registered nurse, I ought to know." I said, "Yes, you should know." "Where did you go to nursing school?" This started a very in-depth conversation about nursing school, where she had worked, what type of nurse she was, etc. In a very short time, she had let go of the hand rails and was very relaxed and talking with me about her career delivering babies.

The above example shows part of the technique I am presenting. Just go with the flow. If someone is trying to go home, walk with them and ask them to describe the home. Ask what color it is, how big it is, who lives there, etc. If someone is upset about a person or animal, ask probing questions to get them to talk about what is happening in his/her head. If someone is angry, find out who or what they are angry about. Generally, you are acknowledging that the person with dementing illness is thinking about something important and that what is important to him/her is important to you. This technique encourages expression of feelings and assists in diminishing behavioral consequences. This technique fosters self-esteem in the person with dementing illness, as well.

What About the Use of Medication?

Many times, sedative, antidepressant, or psychotropic medications are prescribed for persons with dementing illness in an attempt to control agitation, pacing, and aggressiveness. There have been minimal double blind research studies on the effects of these medications on persons with dementia. A major nationwide study for one such drug is underway, and will be years in process before completion.

Clinical research performed at the University of Washington Alzheimer's Disease Research Center is finding use of some of the behavioral interventions previously discussed to be equally as effective, and in some instances more so, than the use of medication in controlling problem behaviors.

My personal experience and that reported by many family members of persons with dementing illness is that medications may make behavior problems worse. Many of these medications cause some dulling of brain responses. This may place the already cognitively impaired person in a situation in which he/she is further cognitively impaired by the drug. However, subjective clinical trials of medications have demonstrated some persons with dementia do respond well to very small doses of some sedatives, antidepressants, or psychotropic drugs. Persons with paranoia or clinical depression particularly may be benefited by appropriate doses of medication.

The best advice I can offer is that if behavior problems are not controlled by methods described in this book or by other behavioral techniques, the caregiver should seek the assistance of a physician specializing in treating behavior problems of persons with dementing illness. Experts in this field who can adequately diagnose and treat specific target behaviors with appropriate amounts of medication may be successful in decreasing or preventing problem behaviors. Furthermore, do not be hesitant, after a very short trial of medication, to contact the prescribing physician to have the medication stopped if behavior problems increase or if the side effects of the medication are worse than the problem it is supposed to prevent.

Additionally, it is important to evaluate any and all medications and combinations (medication interactions) in terms of their effect on cognitive and physical functioning. Anti-Parkinson's medications, for example, may have the opposite effect for which they are intended, causing a decline in cognitive and physical functioning. Also, medications which work well in early stages of dementing illness, may have a negative effect as the disease progresses. A clinical pharmacologist who specializes in evaluating medication effects on the elderly may be the best resource for caregivers who suspect medication effect problems. Consult your physician, as well.

What About Restraints?

I do not recommend the use of physical restraints except in a very critical situation in which the person with dementing illness is harming him/herself or others. I have heard some caregivers say they are practicing the technique of utilizing a loose cloth restraint or a restraint jacket for their loved ones both when in bed and when in a chair. I suppose if your loved one has fallen many times or if he/she can clearly understand and remember why the restraints are there, the utilization of loosely applied cloth restraints may be indicated. However, I would caution you that most people with dementing illness who are not cognizant enough to know they can't walk without assistance, also can't remember why they are finding themselves tied to a bed or a chair. Can you imagine how frightening it would be to find that you are tied down?

If you are caring for someone who wanders, it may be helpful to place a lock higher up on the door so the person can't leave. However, be certain the person is not left alone. If fire broke out, it would be impossible to escape. Generally, I suggest that caregivers not leave their loved ones alone, anyway. Not only is it extremely frightening for the person with dementia to find him/herself alone without a trusted caregiver, but also, undesirable accidents can occur. One member of my support group left the house to run some errands and returned to find his house flooded. His wife had left the kitchen water faucet running and couldn't determine what to do about the problem.

In short, I would encourage you to utilize techniques presented in this book and anything else that works for you to avoid the use of restraints.

Analyzing Behaviors After the Incident

The caregiver needs to attempt to determine the cause of the problem behavior. Frequently the person with dementia has a need that is not being met, and is unable to communicate this need to the caregiver. Thoughtful probing may uncover the problem so the situation can be prevented from occurring in the future. It is important to remember that the person with dementia may not respond to situations in the same way as would someone who has a normally functioning brain. For example, left and right, yes and no, and emotional reactions such as crying or laughter, may be the opposite of what they should be. Careful questioning may uncover the real problem, which may be resolved with minimal changes.

Make every attempt to involve the person with dementing illness in the evaluation process after the emotional response subsides. Not all persons with dementia can respond in a helpful way, but it will save a lot of guessing and trial and error on the part of the caregiver if the person can identify what happened.

I would suggest a method utilized by many behavioral therapists as a framework for analyzing problem behaviors. This framework is frequently referred to as the "ABCs" of behavior evaluation. The letter "A" stands for antecedent, or what happened just prior to the behavior happening. "B" stands for the actual behavior and what happened during the behavior. "C" stands for the consequence of the behavior, or what happened after the behavior occurred. If you are interested in hearing these concepts utilized for many problem behaviors of persons with dementing illness, I have listed, in Appendix A, a series of video tapes available from the University of Washington.

The ABC framework provides a more formal method for evaluating all aspects of problem behaviors. Attempt to find the cause of the behavior. Why do you suppose the person started behaving in this way? The framework further provides a stage for looking at the actual behavior. What happened during the behavior? Finally, it provides a stage for analyzing what happened after the behavior occurred. This final step includes looking at the caregiver and his/her responses, as well as the actual responses of the person with the behavior problem. In other words, what happened to the person as a result of behaving in this way?

Summarizing, managing problem behaviors necessitates the caregiver developing skills of behavior analysis. Observe the behavior over a period of time and make notes about the following:

- How often does the behavior occur?

- When does it happen?

- Where does it happen?

- Who is around when it happens?

- What seems to be triggering the problem?

Then design a plan to minimize or eliminate the behavior problem. Be certain you are not rewarding negative behavior with warmth, kindness, and attention—the act of which will encourage continuing negative behavior.

I again wish to emphasize that utilization of techniques presented throughout this book will go a long way toward preventing problem behaviors. However, if problem behaviors do occur, seek the assistance of a competent medical professional to determine if specific behavioral therapy and/or medication may assist in minimizing the behaviors.

14

MANAGING CONFUSION, DISORIENTATION, AND DEPRESSION

Managing Confusion and Disorientation

It is important to remember that states of confusion and disorientation come and go in the person with dementia. The term *"confusion"* is not a medical term, but is generally utilized to describe someone with muddled thought processes. The term *"disorientation"* refers to the inability to comprehend where one is related to person, time, and place.

We have been led to believe that all persons with dementia are consistently confused, belligerent, and unable to care for themselves. It has been my experience that cognitive abilities of the person with dementia change continually. One minute the person may seem relatively normal, whereas the next minute, hour, or day may be entirely different. It is a major mistake for a caregiver to assume that if the person with dementia cannot understand a concept or perform an activity one minute, hour, day, or week, that he/she always will be unable to perform that activity or function. However, caregivers need to determine when and if a behavior cannot be performed to avoid pushing too hard, the act of which frustrates both the caregiver and overwhelms his/her loved one.

Furthermore, in experiences with my family and friends, what seems like confusion to others or even to me, may not be confusion at all, from the perspective of the person with dementia. For example, frequently after Mother was sleeping at night or napping in the afternoon, she became disoriented as to where she was. She was not able to tell me my name, was shopping in the old market in her home town 40 years ago, or doing something else from the past. She expressed that I was her mother or sister, rather than her daughter. She knew exactly what was happening, but it was at a time and place scores of years ago. By careful verbal cueing and interjecting of appropriate information, she eventually could be brought back to the here and now, so to speak.

This very tedious process is much easier for a family member caregiver who may more easily recognize what the person with dementia is describing, and therefore be able to acknowledge and validate the thoughts of the person with dementia, and then go on to guiding them forward into the present. This process may take anywhere from a few minutes to several hours of occasionally interjecting comments which will move them forward to the present. Additionally, it has been my experience, when talking with persons with dementia, that as they are coming out of a confused state, they express an extreme fear of not knowing what was happening. They are extremely relieved to be back in the present and more reality based. I can't imagine how terrible it must feel to be lost somewhere in a different time and place from the remainder of the world.

I wish to interject some comments about a frequently asked question and/or statement relating to whether or not your loved one knows you. More and more I am objecting to the utilization of the phrase "not knowing." I know my father knew exactly who I was until the day he passed away. He could not express my name, but I could see his eyes light up when I walked into the room. He clearly recognized my presence. Frequently Mother, in her more disoriented states, could not tell me my name. Additionally, sometimes she could not verbalize her name. When she became more lucid and I asked her what was going on in her head when she said she didn't know her name or my name, for example, she invariably indicated she did know who I was and who she was, she just couldn't express her thoughts in words.

Many of my support group members have experienced their loved ones knowing them and responding quite well in situations such as birthday celebrations when they didn't expect any response at all. I feel strongly that we need to assume that our loved ones really do know us and know what is going on around them, but do not have the cognitive ability to verbalize their thoughts. As caregivers, we need to utilize cueing concepts to assist persons with dementing illness to be able to verbalize their thoughts and feelings rather than acting as if they don't know what is happening.

A cardinal mistake of caregivers and others in the presence of someone with dementia who seems confused is that of assuming that the person cannot understand what is being said. I have experienced people in confused states fully comprehending and appropriately responding to simple instructions, and then going back to their "confused" state.

Utilizing the techniques presented throughout this book will assist in minimizing confusion for the person with dementia. However, if the person is disoriented and confused, it is important for the caregiver to give correct information, rather than feeding into the confusion by ignoring the incorrect impressions or agreeing with the incorrect impressions. Honest and gentle guiding toward reality is the most effective means of dealing with the confused person. It is also important for caregivers to deal with feelings which may be expressed during times of confusion or misinterpretation of facts. Caregivers need to be empathetic to the frightening experience the person with dementing illness is enduring. Whatever can be done to assist the person to a more comfortable and oriented state will greatly reduce stress levels and increase cognitive functioning.

Managing Depression

Nearly one third of persons with dementing illness exhibit signs of depression. Significantly, caregivers display symptoms of depression in even higher percentages than do those with dementia. Feelings of sadness, hopelessness, worthlessness, and tearfulness are frequent symptoms. Changes in sleep patterns and eating habits, and losing interest in usual activities are additional symptoms.

The Alzheimer's Disease Research Center at the University of Washington is finding that treating symptoms behaviorally may be more effective than treating with medication in persons with dementing illness. One of the side effects of anti-depressant medication may be a further decline in cognitive functioning.

Additionally, there is some postulation that depression in the person with dementing illness is different from that found in persons without dementia. This difference may explain the ineffectiveness of anti-depressant medications in some of this population. Intuitively, it would seem to me that depression is situation-based in persons with dementia.

Generally, the recommended treatment for those with signs of depression is to utilize many of the techniques previously described in this book. More specifically, effective behavioral techniques follow:

+ Increase the frequency of pleasant events and decrease the frequency of unpleasant events. Look at both social and physical activities that may be pleasant and stimulating. There seems to be a relationship between types of activities and the mood of the person with dementia.

+ Maximize cognitive functioning by utilizing structuring and scheduling techniques described throughout this book.

+ Utilize problem solving techniques to intervene in problem areas.

If utilizing behavioral techniques is ineffective, seek the evaluation of an expert on diagnosis and treatment of depression in persons with dementing illness. Real clinical depression may be effectively treated with anti-depressant medications prescribed in doses appropriate for this population.

I have discussed the moods and reactions of caregivers as they influence the behaviors of persons with dementing illness. Since research is indicating a large percentage of caregivers show signs of depression, it is important for persons providing the care to treat their depression promptly. Utilization of support groups, private counselling, and/or medical treatment may be indicated. Caregivers need to take care of themselves before they can effectively work with persons with dementing illness.

15

PROVIDING A CLIMATE FOR INDEPENDENT FUNCTIONING AND A SENSE OF WELL-BEING

Previous chapters have stressed the importance of promoting independent functioning, both physical and mental, to the highest potential of the person with dementing illness. This section summarizes key concepts for the caregiver to utilize in providing a climate for promoting independence and a sense of well-being.

♦ Provide an environment in which the person with dementia can live with a lifestyle as similar as possible to his/her pre-dementia lifestyle.

♦ Communicate with the person as if he/she understands everything, utilizing techniques described in the section on communicating. If you are having difficulties reaching the person, be creative in your approach. Utilizing pictures and asking the person to point to what he/she wants may work. Maybe a gesture or a squeeze of the hand is all that the person with dementia can generate. Take as much time as is necessary to achieve meaningful communication.

♦ Even though the person may not verbalize appropriate responses, do not assume there is no understanding. The short circuitry in the brain may not allow for appropriate verbal, written, or behavioral responses, but your question or comment may be understood perfectly. Never discuss the person's diminished brain capacity with others in front of the person, assuming he/she will not understand.

♦ Provide enough time in the execution of all physical and intellectual activities for the diseased brain to function without assistance.

♦ Utilize verbal and/or written cueing only if, after allowing enough time for the person to perform the activity independently, there is obvious need for assistance.

♦ Utilize memory stimulating techniques and questions to promote intellectual independence.

♦ Promote relationships and communication (written, verbal, and telephone) with friends and relatives.

♦ Promote a slow-paced, calm, gentle, esteem-building, and supportive atmosphere throughout the day. Give praise such as "good job" or "right," when any physical or intellectual function or part of a function is performed correctly or well.

♦ Display love, affection, nurturing, and touching as appropriate, recognizing the person with dementia may feel insecure, fearful, and very much alone.

* Utilize humor and have a good time with the person with dementing illness. It is very easy to be totally consumed with caregiving. Promote laughter and fun in your therapeutic caregiving environment. Lightening up will reduce the stress levels of both the person with dementia and the caregiver.

* Listen to and make notes of funny comments or actions. As dementia progresses, these notes may help to sustain you through the rough times. Talk a lot about days gone by. You will be amazed at the wealth of information that exudes from the mind of your loved one.

* Remember and recognize the potential for fear and anxiety in the person with dementia, not in performing complex tasks, but in attempting to execute very basic tasks.

* When making decisions regarding a person with dementing illness, always evaluate your alternatives in terms of the potential for increased stress and the degree of adaptability to change that will be required to implement the decision. Minimizing stress and minimizing the need for adaptation to change will keep the person functional both physically and mentally for a longer period of time.

Be aware that a person with dementing illness becomes very dependent upon his/her primary caregiver. A therapeutic caregiver must establish a climate of nurturing and trust. The person dependent on caregiving has to entrust the caregiver with decisions that he/she would normally have made. What a frightening experience it must be to have to entrust someone else to do your thinking and decision making.

Be aware of and considerate of this trust and nurturing position in which you find yourself. Make decisions for the person with dementing illness only if you, as caregiver, have made every attempt to elicit information and decisions from your loved one who has placed his/her trust with you.

16

IS THERAPEUTIC CAREGIVING FOR YOU?

Caring for persons with dementing illness can be challenging, frustrating, and also one of the most rewarding experiences a human being can undertake. Those of us who have been intimately involved in caregiving for loved ones with dementia have found that physical performance as well as mental functioning can be improved through the utilization of many of the techniques described in previous chapters. If expected mental and physical deterioration can be slowed in onset or even reversed somewhat by the use of therapeutic caregiving, the person with dementing illness may live a more active and, hopefully, a better quality of life. This is, to use a cliché, a win-win situation for both the caregiver and the person with dementia.

Maintaining an emotional, physical, and spiritual environment in which the person with dementia can spend his/her waning years with the highest possible quality of life can be immensely rewarding for caregivers. However, I would be the first to admit that the process of caregiving is extremely emotionally and physically exhausting. Not everyone has both the emotional temperament and the physical stamina essential to undertake such a task. Believe me, it takes both!

There is no need to feel guilty if your personal or financial situation does not allow you to be the primary caregiver. I certainly reached a point where it was impossible for me to provide care for my father in his home and he had to go into a convalescent home. Knowing what I have learned since then, I think Dad would have been more functional for a longer period of time if I had been cognizant of some of the techniques presented in this book. I know, however, I did the best I could with the knowledge I had at the time.

If you do choose to keep your loved one in your home, and you need to employ caregivers to assist you, this alternative may be more expensive than paying for care in a nursing home. Many people have the financial resources to handle this major expense. Others do not.

The Need for Caregiver Respite

If the decision is to maintain the person with dementing illness in the family home, it will become more and more important for the primary caregiver to have some sort of respite. This need is equally important for family member caregivers such as spouses, sons, or daughters, and for employed in-home caregivers. No human being is capable of maintaining the constant keenness and intensity of mental attention or the constant level of physical assistance that is required in caring for a person with dementia day in and day out, week in and week out. During early phases of the dementia causing illness, one person may be able to manage emotionally and physically for extended periods. As the dementing process continues, however, there will be increasing need for some sort of total break, away from the caregiving environment.

Fortunately, many respite options are available to caregivers that were unheard of when I started this process in 1981. I realize these options may be available only in major metropolitan centers, however.

One option is that of adult day centers. There are several types of centers. Some provide an entire array of professionals including nurses, social workers, physical and occupational therapists, and activity coordinators. These centers may be designated as day health centers. Others do not offer this assortment of health services. Some are available only one or two days a week. Others are available daily. Some are a part of a nursing home or Alzheimer's Care Center. Others are free standing in different locations in the community. All provide meals and an assortment of planned activities to keep the person with dementing illness active and involved. These centers work best for people who are not afraid of groups of people and who can adapt somewhat to a change in physical environment and numerous staff. People in more advanced stages of dementing illness usually are not accepted in these centers. Furthermore, many persons with dementia are not able to adapt to the change in physical environment and to the need to socialize with many people in a group setting. People I have observed at adult day centers seem to be enjoying their time and express looking forward to attending. Fortunately, the trend is toward longer hours to meet the needs of working family member caregivers and exhausted caregivers who need respite.

Overnight respite is frequently available in adult family homes, nursing homes, Alzheimer's disease units, or assisted living units. Length of stay varies with the particular facility. Some allow stays of up to two weeks. Others, only allow a maximum of two days.

Another option for some may be to do what I did with Mother. I cared for her in my home, with some employed assistance, for several months following her major stroke in 1988. Then I placed her in a loving and caring convalescent facility part time. The remainder of the time she was at my home. We worked with extensive exercising, cueing, and social stimulation that she did not receive in the institutional living environment. I would have loved to have had Mother here with me on a full time basis. I found, however, with my perfectionistic personality and my need for privacy and alone time, that I could not tolerate having employed caregivers in my home on an ongoing basis. I felt my privacy was being invaded, and I rarely got the respite I needed even with someone employed to care for Mom. Since Mother needed 24 hour a day care, the only alternative for me was the one I have described. Mother fully understood and was appreciative of the opportunities to come to my home as frequently as she did.

Family member caregivers may find that employing respite caregivers is the most convenient way to break away from constant caregiving. The person with dementing illness will not have a need to adapt to a strange physical environment or to interact with many new people in this type of respite setting. Some caregivers prefer to have someone with their loved ones at night to ensure a full night of sleep. Others prefer to have someone available during the day, freeing the caregiver to leave the home and socialize and/or run errands. Many prefer a complete break for 24 or 48 hours weekly. The primary caregiver must determine the times, frequency, and hours which will best meet his/her needs for rest and relaxation.

If an in-home caregiver is hired, don't assume he/she has appropriate training to provide therapeutic care. Very few people working in home health agencies or in long term care environments are trained in therapeutic caregiving techniques. Check carefully for the employed caregiver's philosophy of care. It may be more important to find someone who is inexperienced and eager to learn, has a pleasant personality and possesses common sense, and train him/her yourself, rather than to "try to teach an old dog new tricks."

It is important, if family members hire caregivers, to recognize that these employed caregivers need respite and/or private time, as well. As the dementia process increases, it is impossible for one person to provide live-in assistance on a round-the-clock basis. Even in early stages, it is important for live-in caregivers to have one or two days off a week. No one working with persons with dementing illness can maintain his/her mental equilibrium without planned, scheduled relief. Most of us are used to a forty hour work week. We need to remember that caregiving is a non-stop proposition for 24 hours out of every day. None of us has the physical stamina or the emotional tolerance to maintain the sharp edge needed to provide therapeutic caregiving without frequent breaks.

What If You Must Move Your Loved One?

If therapeutic caregiving is what you desire for your loved one, do not expect the kind of care discussed in this book to be provided in an institutional setting, whether it be a retirement home, assisted living unit, nursing home, an Alzheimer's Unit, or an adult family home or group home. Simply stated, the type of therapeutic caregiving discussed in this book usually requires a 1:1 ratio of caregivers to persons with dementing illness. The reality of staffing ratios of actual caregivers to residents in institutions may be anywhere from 1:8 up to 1:25 depending on the shift and/or the facility in which your loved one may be placed. This statement is not meant to be a criticism of the hard work of caregivers and the loving and nurturing care given in many institutions. It is merely an objective statement of the reality of care in institutional settings.

If you are not able to provide for care of your loved one in his/her familiar environment, it is important to carefully consider options available. Frequently, those responsible are so anxious to be relieved of this tremendous caregiving burden that unwise decisions are made. Following are some tips for making appropriate placement decisions.

◆   When possible, respect the wishes of the person with dementing illness. I encourage caregivers to discuss the caregiving dilemma with their loved ones if at all possible. If impending dementia decline is discussed and proper planning is done early on, it will be much easier to make the appropriate decisions and the ultimate move when the time comes. Many couples or family members make commitments to each other not to place the other in a nursing home. Of course, none of us would leap at the chance to go into a nursing home or any other out-of-home caregiver situation. The request can be acknowledged, but we must recognize that usually when persons make these pacts not to institutionalize the other, they are in good health and of sound mind. However, when the situation changes, as in the case of dementing illness, most people see the need for these pacts to be broken.

My parents are a good example of this type of situation. Not only did they promise each other they would not place the other in a nursing home, they also stated over and over again that if they became disabled they did not want their children to take care of them. However, as first Dad, and then Mother became more and more disabled with dementing illness, both of their positions changed. Mother could well understand the need to place Dad in a facility when the time arose. She and I combed the area to find the best placement for him. As Mom declined, she was more than pleased that I became very involved in her care. Although she felt I had given up too much of my life for her and Dad, she welcomed my presence, and thanked me frequently.

If you must move your loved one and you are meeting resistance, be firm, but caring in your response. Use touch and nurturing to reassure your loved one. Make plans to be with your loved one in the new environment for several weeks to ease the transition. Do not attempt to make arrangements with your loved one by telephone. Be there to offer firm, but caring support. Do not get into a spiraling argumentative situation with your loved one. Trying to be rational does not get through to someone with dementing illness in an agitated state. Remember, the agitation is probably due to fear—fear of going into a new environment and fear of separation from, in many cases, a life long love, companion, or family member, or at least a trusted caregiver and/or a familiar environment. If he/she is getting upset, wait a bit and try a new approach.

So, respect the wishes of your loved one if at all possible to do so. If not, do the best you can to placed your loved one in a caring facility.

- Plan ahead to search for appropriate facility(s) and care. Frequently families are in a crisis when they make the decision to move their loved one. It is much better to plan ahead if at all possible. Early on, visit facilities in your neighborhood and determine what they have to offer. There are many booklets available from government agencies describing how to choose a nursing home or other facility. Chapters in some books in the Complementary Reading List in Appendix A cover this topic, as well.

- If you are making decisions in a crisis situation, plan ahead from where you are in time. Remember that no matter what is happening at present, dementing illness will continue to cause a decline in functioning. What may seem appropriate currently, may not suffice in the future. I am not suggesting that you move someone directly from home to a nursing home. Rather I am suggesting that you choose an entry facility that allows for increased care without having to make another major move. Frequently assisted living units can suffice initially. If the assisted living unit is physically connected to or coordinated with an Alzheimer's unit, a special care unit, or a nursing home, the transition will be much easier for your loved one.

- Look for facilities that have an atmosphere of caring and human warmth. Are residents clean and well kept? Does the facility look and smell clean? Would you consider placing yourself in such a facility. When Mother and I were looking, we found vast differences. I reviewed state nursing home survey reports as one method for limiting the scope of my search. There seemed to be a high correlation between what looked like a good facility from a lay point of view and what was found in survey reports. Use your intuitive judgment.

- If you must move your loved one, ignore the request of the facility to stay away for a week or two. Some facilities seem to think people adapt better if there is no contact with family members or previous caregivers. However, as an advocate for persons with dementing illness, I can't imagine anything much more cruel than to remove the person from a familiar environment and caregivers into a totally strange physical environment and strange people and prohibit contact with familiar people. A forced separation may be very cruel to the family member caregiver, as well. Former caregivers should stay with the person with dementing illness as much as is possible, assisting the person to adapt to this very strange world. Adaptation may take up to two months.

- If you are geographically distant from your loved one, unless there are strong family ties to the area in which your loved one resides, it may be preferable to move your loved one to a facility near you. I found it nearly impossible to provide appropriate supervision and assistance when my parents were only two and a half hours away. It is impossible to do so with longer distances. I feel it is essential for someone, preferably a caring family member, to make frequent (daily, or minimally weekly) **evaluatory** visits to the facility in which your loved one resides. One would like to think that if you placed your loved one in a facility designed to care for the elderly that everything will go well. The reality of institutional life, however, is that it is impossible for facilities to either continually evaluate or meet the needs of your loved one placed there. Once again, I am not being critical of the many facilities and their staff who do their best to provide quality care and meet resident needs. I am merely stating the facts of institutional life.

If you are unable to move your loved one close to you, and have no family member who can be responsible for supervision and evaluation of care, I would suggest you employ an elder care specialist to provide this service for you. The National Association of Professional Geriatric Care Managers, head quartered in Tucson, Arizona, provides a country-wide listing of specialists in this area. The phone number for this organization is (602) 881-8008.

If you, as a caregiver/decision maker for a person with dementing illness, are able to provide the choice between employed caregivers in the person's home versus moving to another facility consider first and foremost the amount of change and consequent adaptation that will be required. Previous chapters on stress and problem behaviors as well as others provide information on the difficulties with coping with environmental or people changes. Given the financial wherewithal and/or the emotional and physical stamina of caregivers, it will be considerably easier for the person with dementing illness to be provided with therapeutic care in his/her familiar environment.

Therapeutic caregiving in a familiar environment will not only assist the person to be mentally and physically more functional for a longer period, but will also improve the quality of life for the person with dementing illness. The quality of life of loving family members will be enhanced in so doing.

Remember, therapeutic family member caregiving is an extremely demanding and grueling responsibility. Again, I am referring to caregiving in the broadest sense. Whether you are a geographically distant son or daughter with moral and financial responsibility for your loved one, or an on site loving and caring spouse, the burden, in terms of responsible decision making, is the same. I sincerely hope this book will guide you in making appropriate decisions both for you and for your loved one with dementing illness.

If you do choose to provide some or all of the on site caregiving, I wish you well in your endeavors. Rarely in life will you have the opportunity to provide this type of devoted and sustaining care for a loved one. The extreme demands, if you are emotionally and physically strong enough to meet them, are outweighed by the emotional closeness you attain in caring for your loved one. Many people ask me if I would make the same decisions regarding my involvement if I were to be making the decisions today. My response, without hesitation, is "yes."

AFTERWORD

Mother passed away November 16, 1995, after finally reaching the point where she could no longer swallow, and contracting aspiration pneumonia. During the last few hours of her life, as I was sitting by her bedside holding her hand, I felt compelled to write a letter to her, professing her many attributes and telling her how much I loved her. Several of my friends and colleagues have encouraged me to incorporate that letter in this slightly revised second printing of my book.

At first I felt the letter was too personal to share publicly. However, as I am reading it now, with tears in my eyes two months since Mother's passing, I realize the feeling tones projected in the letter may have value to some readers of this book. The letter follows for your perusal.

Thursday, November 16th, 2:00 p.m.

Dear Mom:

I'm sitting by your bedside as you slowly slip away, knowing there is fairly little I can do for you now except to try my best to keep you from suffering as you face life's final journey. You are facing this difficult time in your usual style—with tenacity, straight-forwardness, caring, concern, and a little dab of humor.

I couldn't believe, when I was called to your bedside Tuesday evening, that as sick and exhausted as you were, you managed to tell me you were "sorry I was sick." (I had a severe bronchitis with a high fever.) I knew I could clear those secretions out of your lungs and make your breathing easier, but when I asked, you told me, "No." When I asked if you were tired and wanted to slip away, you nodded your head, "Yes." Although I felt helpless, I respected your decision, because I knew that even as your life ebbs, you have the same infinite wisdom, and decisive, practical approach to life that you so ably passed on to Byron and to me. I am tremendously thankful you were able to make the choice yourself, and you were and continue to be at peace with your decision. I will always remember your last big smile and little chuckle when I placed your big, gray, floppy-eared stuffed bunny on your bed where you could see her.

As I reflect back over 55 years of life together, for some reason or other, I don't remember a lot about my early childhood. I do remember when I was awakening from ether anesthetic after Dr. Klein yanked out my tonsils, you were asking him if I could have ice cream to soothe my sore throat. Well, mother, I don't know if that was the moment I learned to like ice cream, but to this day, it is one of my favorite foods. I remember you making your favorite peach ice cream the old-fashioned rock salt and ice way at the bottom of the back porch at our home in Orillia. What a major project, but then you always provided us with wonderful food—all made from "scratch" with fresh ingredients, and always served when everyone in the family was appropriately seated at the table. In fact, I remember how astonished and uncomfortable some of my high school friends were in having to actually sit at a table to eat, and even more so, to stay there until every one in the family finished eating. Yours and Dad's warm welcome and your scrumptious food, however, soon made them feel at ease.

I also remember your compassion for animals. You treated our farm animals like people. Some of my fondest childhood memories are of trips to the Woodland Park Zoo and Mount Rainier, where it was obvious you had a special connection with wildlife. My most precious pictures are those of you feeding the deer and chipmunks. Your wildlife connection never left, as I have had the more recent joy of watching you observe birds and squirrels in my back yard. The last day you were home, November 6th, on your 91st Birthday, you were watching one of your bushy-tailed friends, and even though you weren't responding to much of anything else, you became more alert when I brought you your little bunny, "Muffy."

Your love for flowers and all growing things was evident in your beautiful flower gardens. How I have enjoyed, in these last few years, our annual trips to the Skagit Valley to look at the tulips, and driving around the countryside looking for fall leaf color. How appropriate that the fall leaf color here this year has been the best I have seen since returning to the Northwest. I am grateful that we had the opportunity to share in such a colorful display of nature in your last fall season.

As I look back on my years of growing up, I remember how you always made things happen. Your extreme organizational skills and solid leadership traits provided an essential sense of structure. Home was always a safe and secure haven for me. You were always available and doing things for us kids. You always encouraged us to climb the next step on the ladder, and you always praised us along the way. From keeping a meticulously clean house and manicured yard, to assisting us with homework and carting us all over the place to 4-H and school activites, everything always seemed to get done and done on time. And you always had time to meet special needs.

I have always been in awe of your extreme intelligence, and especially of your cleverness—a gene carrying the latter you did not pass on to me. I fondly remember, when I was running for student body offices at Renton High School, and had been racking my feeble brain for weeks trying to come up with campaign slogans, that when I asked you for assistance, you rattled off one-liners non-stop, while standing at the ironing board working on Dad's shirts. By the way, you didn't pass on your baby soft skin gene to me either.

It was our last several years together that I remember with most fondness. Our closeness grew as we were faced first with the difficult times with Dad, and then as we worked together facing the devastating process of you slowly losing your brain functions. I kick myself periodically for not having had the sense to keep a journal of our experiences together, but a few incidents come to mind as I reflect back on these past few years.

I have loving memories of our trip to Denmark, Scotland, and England in 1983. After having been sick the early part of the summer, I remember how hard you worked to get yourself in physical shape to endure the trip. You were your usual hard-driven self as we traipsed from place to place, in and out of subway tunnels, and on and off busses and trains. Remember how scared you were when we got in the car in Scotland during evening rush hour and you realized I was going to be driving "on the wrong side of the road?"

As your ability to communicate dwindled, I have so reveled in your funny quips or astute statements. I guess I always was aware of how proud you were to be Danish because you occasionally would remark that you raised children that weren't Danish enough to drink coffee. I remember one day about a year ago that I left you and your favorite breakfast companion, Honey Bear, to finish your coffee. When I returned I asked if you and your bear had finished your coffee. You retorted with perfect timing, "Not this bear, he isn't Danish."

I also vividly remember an evening when we had a few relatives and friends for dinner. You had not participated in any conversation throughout the meal, but I sensed you were following the discussion. I asked one of our guests, a super salesman with a gift of gab a mile long to sit with you while we cleared the table and prepared dessert. This gentlemen, in his usual style, started making effusive comments about you—your silver hair, your intelligence, etc. All of a sudden you said, "You describe me perfectly." This from you, my most modest and humble mother. I nearly dropped a handful of dishes.

My proudest moment in life was when I had just completed my book earlier this year and I was telling you I had written a book. I asked if you would like to guess the subject. You responded, "I hope it is about taking care of people like me." That was the longest sentence I had hear you speak in more than a year, Mother. I shall always remember this most gracious and grateful comment.

As we have worked together as a team these past few years, me filling in the gaps for your ever-increasing loss of brain function, we have become closer and closer. As your ability to communicate dwindled, my ability increased. We are such kindred spirits, Mother, I am certain you can feel and understand the content of this letter, as I watch you fading from me and going to a peaceful and restful place to be with Dad. I know I have told you over and *over, but I do so hope that you can sense my deep love for you. I know you will have a special place in Heaven.*

With everlasting love,

Barbara

P.S. I am sorry I left you for about 15 minutes in the middle of writing this letter, Mother, but I went out to get an ice cream cone to soothe my aching heart. I kept the base of the cone to give to your little bunny, Muffin. I will always remember how you loved to give her the base of your ice cream cone, and watch her delight and hear the crunching as she devoured it and then jumped up and down with ears flopping. Don't forget our little memory-stimulating jingle, Mother—"I know a little bunny and her name is Muffy, and a very good friend is she..."

I sincerely hope you have not been bored with this personal accounting of life with Mother. I do hope that the letter projects the many positive aspects of caring for persons with dementing illness. Along with the tremendously grueling emotional and physical aspects of caregiving, there can be many deep-seated rewards. My best to you in your caregiving endeavors.

APPENDIX A: COMPLEMENTARY RESOURCE LIST

I have selected a few readings and video tapes which I feel best complement the content of this book. This list is not intended to be an all-inclusive listing of resources on caring for persons with dementing illness. Many of the following books have complete bibliographies which will assist you if you wish to seek further information.

Complementary Reading List

- Bergquist, William H., Rod McLean, and Barbara A. Kobylinski. *Stroke Survivors*. San Francisco: Jossey-Bass Publishers, 1994. 261 pp.

- Carter, Rosalynn, and Susan K. Golant. *Helping Yourself Help Others—A Book for Caregivers*. New York: Times Books, Random House., 1994. 278 pp.

- Cohen, Donna, Ph.D., and Carol Eisdorfer, Ph.D., M.D. *The Loss of Self, A Family Resource for the Care of Alzheimer's Disease and Related Disorders*. New York: NAL Penguin, Inc., 1986. 377 pp.

♦   Coughlan, Patricia Brown. *Facing Alzheimer's, Family Caregivers Speak.* New York: Ballantine Books, 1993. 261 pp.

♦   Feil, Naomi, ACSW. *V/F Validation: The Feil Method.* Cleveland, Ohio: Edward Feil Productions, 1992. 130 pp.

To order contact: Edward Feil Productions, 4616 Prospect Avenue, Cleveland Ohio, 44103.

♦   Gruetzner, Howard, M.Ed. *Alzheimer's, A Caregiver's Guide and Sourcebook.* New York: John Wiley and Sons, Inc., 1992. 308 pp.

♦   Lustbader, Wendy and Nancy R. Hooyman. *Taking Care of Aging Family Members, A Practical Guide.* New York: The Free Press, 1994. 356 pp.

♦   Lustbader, Wendy. *Counting on Kindness, The Dilemmas of Dependency.* New York: The Free Press, 1991. 206 pp.

♦   Mace, Nancy L., M.A., and Peter V. Rabins, M.D., M.P.H. *The 36 Hour Day.* New York: Warner Books, Inc., 1991. 412 pp.

♦   Perkins-Carpenter, Betty. *How to Prevent Falls.* New York: St. Martin's Press, 1991. 100 pp.

♦   Richards, Marty. "Meeting the Spiritual Needs of the Cognitively Impaired," *Generations,* Fall 1990, 63-64.

♦   Rob, Caroline, R.N., and Janet Reynolds, G.N.P. *The Caregiver's Guide, Helping Elderly Relatives Cope with*

Health and Safety Problems. Boston: Houghton Mifflin Company, 1991. 458 pp.

♦ Robinson, Anne and Beth Spencer and Laurie White. *Understanding Difficult Behaviors, Some Practical Suggestions for Coping with Alzheimer's Disease and Related Illnesses.* Ypsilanti, Michigan: Eastern Michigan University, 1992. 80 pp.

To order contact: Alzheimer's Care and Training Center, Senior Health Building, 5401 McAuley Drive, P.O. Box 994, Ann Arbor, MI 48106.

Phone: (313) 572-4334

♦ Sherman, James R., Ph.D. *Preventing Caregiver Burnout.* (Plus entire caregiver series). Golden Valley, Minnesota: Pathway Books, 1994. 80pp.

To order contact: Pathway Books, 700 Parkview Terrace, Golden Valley, MN 55416-3439.

Phone: (612) 377-1512

♦ Task Force on Aging. (3 publications) *How to Hire Helpers, Reclaiming Time: Caregiver Relief and Renewal,* and *Time to Decide (end of life decisions)* Seattle: Church Council of Greater Seattle, 1991, 1996.

To order contact: Church Council Task Force on Aging, 4759 - 15th Avenue N.E., Seattle, WA 98105.

Phone: (206) 525-1213

- *Wiser Now,* Newsletter. Waquiot, Massachusetts Better Directions, Inc.

  Available from Better Directions, P.O. Box 3064, Waquoit, MA, 02536-3064.

  Phone: (800) 999-0795

Video Tape Resources

- Series of 5 tapes from the Alzheimer's Disease and Related Disorders Association, Inc. Cover many aspects of caring for persons with dementing illness. A good broad perspective. Done with feeling and sensitivity. Check with your local Alzheimer's Association office. For further information contact:

  Alzheimer's Disease and Related Disorders Association, Inc., 919 North Michigan Avenue, Suite 100, Chicago, Illinois 60611-1676.

  Phone: (800) 272-3900

- Behavior management tapes from the University of Washington Alzheimer's Disease Research Center. Narrated by Linda Teri, Ph.D. Behavior evaluation techniques. Tapes may be available through local Alzheimer's Association office. If not, contact:

University of Washington, Alzheimer's Disease Research Center, University of Washington Department of Psychiatry, XD-43, Seattle, Washington 98195.

Phone: (206) 543-6761

◆ Sit and Be Fit™ exercise and equipment video tape series. Toning and stretching exercises which may be suitable in early stages of dementia. For further information contact:

Sit and Be Fit, Inc., P.O. Box 8033, Spokane, WA 99201-0033

Phone: (509) 449-9438

Dementia Information and Support Groups

◆ Alzheimer's Disease and related dementia-causing diseases:

Contact your local chapter usually found in the white pages of your telephone directory, or contact the national association:

Alzheimer's Disease and Related Disorders Association, Inc., 919 North Michigan Avenue, Suite 100 Chicago, Illinois 60611-1676.

Phone: (800) 272-3900

Internet Address: http://www.alz.org/

◆   Parkinson's Disease:

National Parkinson's Foundation
1501 N.W. Ninth Aveune
Miami, Florida 33136

Phone: (800) 327-4545

◆   Stroke Association:

National Stroke Association
8450 East Orchard Road, Suite 1000
Englewood, Colorado 80111-5015

Phone: (800) STROKES   787-6537

APPENDIX B:
SAMPLE DAILY SCHEDULE

Note:

This is merely a sample. Actual activities appropriate to the condition and needs of your person with dementia should be specifically indicated on the schedule. Make in large format and post in easily observed place. Give your loved one control of his/her schedule if at all possible.

TIME	ACTIVITY
7:00 am	Get up—orient to day; set out clothes; toilet; shower or bath; shave; oral hygiene; dress
8:00 am	Breakfast—encourage fluids; oral hygiene; toilet for B.M.; make bed; empty trash
9:00 am	Read paper; discuss world events
9:30 am	Morning exercise—warm-up, range-of-motion balance, and stretching every day except Sunday; aerobic exercise—Monday, Wednesday, Friday; toning exercises—Tuesday, Thursday, Saturday

10:00 am   Toilet; fluids; snack, if appropriate; oral hygiene

11:00 am   Mind stimulating activities—math, spelling, counting, puzzles, writing, reading, etc.

12:00 noon   Toilet; lunch—encourage fluids; oral hygiene; toilet after lunch, cue for B.M. if none after breakfast

1:00 pm   Afternoon rest period

2:00 pm   Toilet; walk or other activity

3:00 pm   Fluids; relaxing activity such as letter writing, telephoning, etc.

4:00 pm   Toilet; mind stimulating activity

5:00 pm   Toilet; dinner—encourage fluids; oral hygiene; toilet after dinner, cue for B.M. if none after break fast or lunch

6:00 pm   Relaxing activity

8:00 pm   Toilet; snack, if appropriate; oral hygiene

9:00 pm   Toilet; shower, if necessary; ready for bed

APPENDIX C:
SAMPLE ORAL HYGIENE
CUEING REGIMEN

ORAL HYGIENE CUEING

- Rinse mouth with water

- Squish hard

- Spit it out

- Use Stimudents between top teeth

- Use Stimudents between bottom teeth

- Floss upper teeth—evening only

- Floss lower teeth—evening only

- Place toothpaste on brush

- Brush 10 counts on outside left top

- Brush 10 counts on outside left bottom

- Brush 10 counts on front top

- Brush 10 counts on front bottom

- Brush 10 counts on outside right top

- Brush 10 counts on outside right bottom

- Brush 25 counts on inside top

- Brush 25 counts on inside bottom

- Rinse brush and put away

- Rinse mouth with water

- Squish hard

- Spit it out

- Rise mouth with mouthwash

- Squish hard

- Spit it out

- Rinse out glass

- Put glass away

APPENDIX D:
SAMPLE CUEING REGIMEN FOR GETTING OUT OF A CHAIR OR OFF A TOILET SEAT

- Scoot bottom out to the edge of chair

- Get belly even with edge of seat

- Place feet back

- Place feet shoulder width apart

- Place hands on chair arms (if any)

- Lean forward

- Nose over toes

- Push up and forward

- Pull bottom forward and stand up tall

Note: Caregiver needs to place hands on front of body if he/she wants the person to lean or push forward. If hands are placed on the back of the body, the person will lean backward, not forward.

APPENDIX E1:
INTRODUCTION TO EXERCISE
SEGMENTS

General Information

These exercises are designed to be safe and effective if instructions are followed carefully. **Please check with your physician before starting any exercise program.**

All of these exercise segments are designed for persons who have enough strength and stamina to stand and exercise. They are or can be adapted to using a counter edge or chair back as a stabilizing mechanism if free-standing balance is a problem. If you are working with someone who cannot stand and exercise, please contact me at (800) 799-3414 to discuss your particular needs. I have exercise sets available, for a minimal fee, for persons who are confined to a chair and for those who have had a stroke or other paralyzing conditions.

Exercise Frequency

As discussed in Chapter 9 in more detail, daily exercise of some type should be routinely scheduled. Warm up, stretching, range of motion, and balance exercises should be performed daily—or at least 5 days a week. Aerobic activity should be performed minimally 3 times a week, spread throughout the week. Daily aerobic activity will not only assist in promoting heart and lung conditioning and improving circulation, but also, reduce stress levels. Working with weights should be performed 3 times a week, with a day of rest between sessions. Stretching and cool down exercises should be performed after both aerobic exercise and working with weights.

Appropriate Clothing

Clothing should be loose, stretchable, and comfortable in feel as well as in warmth. Dress warmly enough when outdors for activities such as walking. On warm days, dress cooly enough to encourage movement. When exercising inside, dress with loosely fitting clothing to encourage necessary movement.

Shoes must be durable and have appropriate support for walking and exercising. I recommend the use of a good pair of non-skid sole walking shoes or fitness/athletic shoes. Shoes must tie in place for stability. Socks should be absorbent in nature. A good pair of athletic socks can be worn over women's hosiery during exercise sessions.

The Importance of Counting

Encourage the person with dementing illness to count exercise repetions out loud. Counting will provide mental stimulation and promote thinking.

APPENDIX E2:
WARM-UP, BALANCE, RANGE OF MOTION, AND STRETCHING EXERCISES

NOTE: **DO NOT UNDERTAKE ANY TYPE OF EXERCISE ACTIVITY WITHOUT APPROVAL OF YOUR PHYSICIAN!**

Warm-Up and Balance Exercises

Frequency: Daily (5-6 days per week)

When: Before aerobic exercise or toning exercises

Warm up exercises are important to prevent injury to muscles when exercising. They are designed to get the blood circulating at a more intense level throughout the body. With better circulation, the muscles warm up and can be pulled and stretched further without injury. **Warm up exercises should be done before beginning any type of exercise activity, including walking.**

➤ Sideways Stepping:

Step sideways to the right, swinging arms toward the right and up. Step sideways to the left, swinging arms toward the left and up. Gradually increase reach of arms outward and upward. Do not reach above shoulder height. Continue swinging for 1 minute.

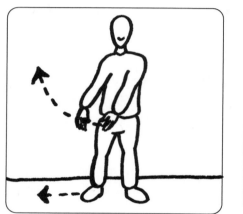
Right

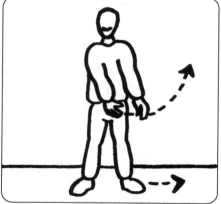
Left

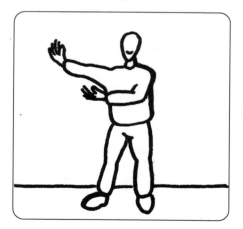
Progressing Right

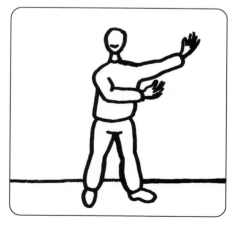
Progressing Left

➤ Marching:

March in place or around room for approximately 1 minute. Lift knees as high as is comfortable, **but not above waist height.** Land on your toes and roll through to your heels. Swing arms naturally at side. Gradually increase arm movements. Pump hard with your arms if you can.

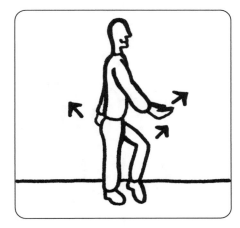

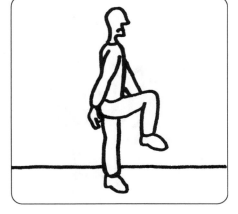

Correct   Incorrect

➤ Upward Reaching:

Stand with feet shoulder width apart. Reach arms overhead, and slightly forward **in full view of eyes to prevent back injury.** Stretch upward a little farther first with the right hand and then with the left hand. Do 3 repetitions. Right stretch + left stretch = 1 repetition.

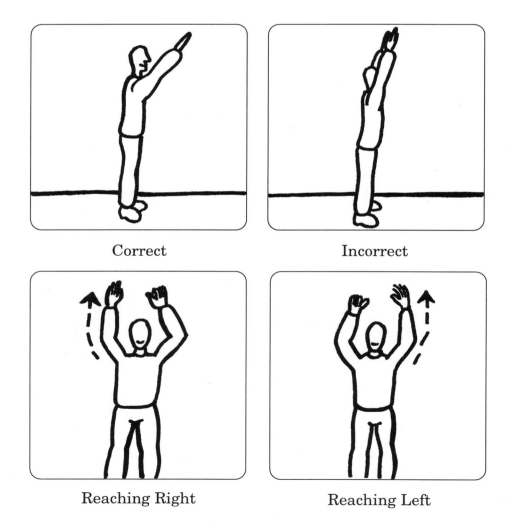

Correct	Incorrect

Reaching Right	Reaching Left

➤ Side Stretches:

Stand with feet shoulder width apart. Keep right arm down and reach overhead with left arm. **With upright posture, looking sideways over your shoulder**, bend right to stretch your left side, bringing your left arm over your head in a "C" shape. Hold stretch for a count of 5. Repeat, reaching up and over with your right arm.

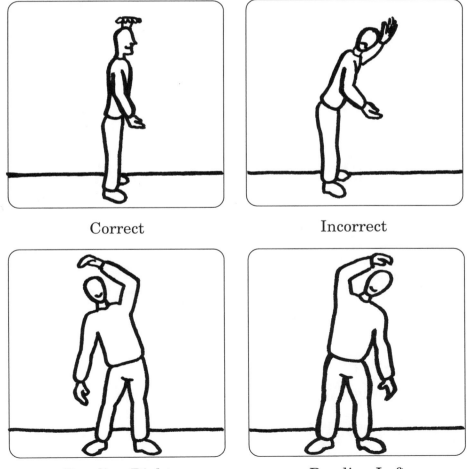

Correct   Incorrect

Bending Right   Bending Left

➤ Leg Stretches:

Stand with feet shoulder width apart, using counter top or chair back for hand support if necessary, step back with right foot, keeping right leg almost straight. Your left knee will bend. **Be certain your feet are placed in such a way that your left knee does not go beyond your toes to protect your knee. Keep trunk in upright position.** Place heel of right foot on the floor and hold to a count of 5. Move right foot forward. Step back with the left foot and hold to a count of 5.

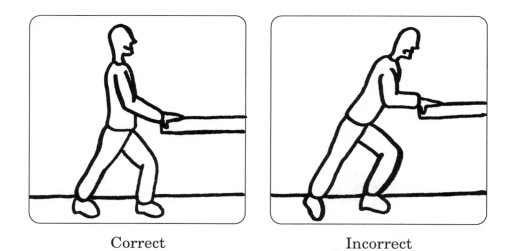

Correct   Incorrect

➤ Repeat above exercise with each leg, taking your hands away from the chair back or counter top for as long as you can—up to a count of 5.

➤ One Leg Balance:

Stand with your feet slightly apart in front of counter top or
sturdy chair back. Hold counter top or chair back for support
if necessary. Standing erect, lift right foot off floor with foot
hanging straight down. Hold for a count of 5. Repeat, without
holding hand support if possible.

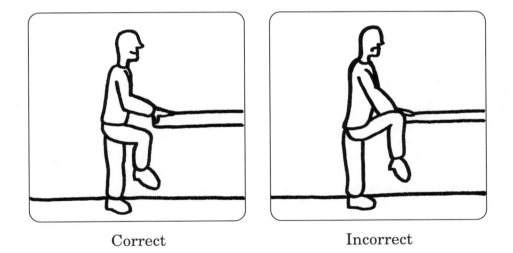

Correct   Incorrect

➤ Repeat above exercise lifting left foot off of floor.

Range of Motion Exercises

Frequency: Daily and whenever you feel like moving.

When: After warm-up and balancing exercises.

Range of motion exercises keep all joints and muscles function-ing to their fullest capacity. Without working joints and muscles within their full range of movement, they become stiff and in-flexible, making normal movements and performing daily activi-ties more difficult. You may choose to do them either standing or sitting in a straight-backed chair with no arms or on a stool or bench.

A note to caregivers:

It is important to let the person do as much as is possible on his/her own. However, being able to perform a full range of movement in each of the exercises is crucial to maintaining joint mobility. If the person with dementing illness is not getting a full range of motion without assistance, do at least 5 of each of the repetitions with your assistance. **Never force a joint or muscle to move—just do slow, gentle, and firm movements.**

If the person with dementing illness has not been physically active, particularly in using all muscle groups, he/she will have to build up to the recommended number of 10 repetitions. For the first two weeks do 3 repetitions. The third and fourth weeks,

do 6 repetitions. The fifth week, do 10 repetitions unless otherwise indicated on the specific exercise.

➤ Head Up and Down:

Either sitting or standing, with your head centered on your
body, and your arms hanging straight down and your shoulders relaxed, move your head slowly and gently up and down,
alternately letting your chin fall clear to your chest and tipping your nose up toward the ceiling just looking up toward
the ceiling with your eyes. **Be certain your head is not
tipped to one side when doing this exercise. Do not
hyperextend your neck by tipping your head back too
far.** Build to 10 repetitions.

➤ Head Turning Side to Side:

Either sitting or standing, with your head centered on your
body, and your arms hanging straight down and your shoulders relaxed, **slowly and gently** turn your head and look
behind your right shoulder. Look as far behind you as you
can. Then turn your head and look behind your left shoulder.
**Be certain your head is not tipped to one side when
doing this exercise. Do not look upward when doing
this exercise.** Right side + left side = one repetition. Build
to 10 repetitions.

➤ Head Tipping Side to Side:

Sitting or standing, with your head centered on your body, and your arms hanging straight down, pushing toward the floor with the heel of your hands (shoulders pushing down-ward), **slowly and gently** tip the top of your head toward your right shoulder as far as it will go. **Do not pull your shoulder up to your ear. Do not look upward.** Then, tip your head toward the left shoulder. Right tip + left tip = one repetition. Build up to 10 repetitions.

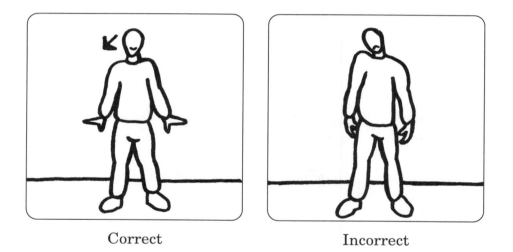

Correct   Incorrect

➤ Neck Stretching:

Either sitting or standing, pushing down toward the floor with the heel of your hands (shoulders pushing downward), tip your head to put your chin on your chest. Turn your head slightly to the right. Let your head hang down, with your left ear reaching toward your left breast. Count to 5. Bring your head to an upright position. Put your chin back on your chest. Turn your head slightly to the left. Let your head hang down, with your right ear reaching toward your right breast. Count to 5. Do one repetition only.

➢ Shoulder Shrugs:

Either sitting or standing, raise your shoulders up toward your head, then push your shoulders down. If you can't get your two shoulders coordinated to work at the same time, do each individually. Build up to 10 repetitions.

➢ Shoulders, Forward Circles:

Preferably standing, with feet shoulder width apart and arms straight and slightly away from your body, and your palms facing downward, make forward circles with your arms rotating from the shoulder. Make as big a circle as is comfortable. If you can't get your two arms coordinated, do each individually. Build up to 10 circles.

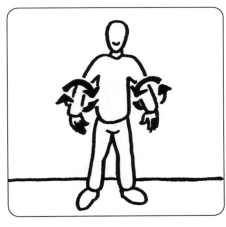
Correct

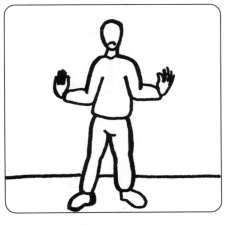
Incorrect

➤ Shoulders, Backward Circles:

Preferably standing, with your feet shoulder width apart and your arms hanging straight down, and elbows straight, and your palms facing forward toward the front of your body, make backward circles with your arms. Make as big a circle as is comfortable. If you can't get your two arms coordinated to work at the same time, do each individually. Build up to 10 circles.

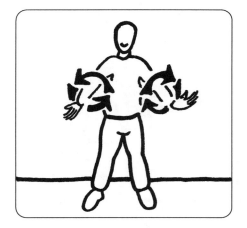

Correct

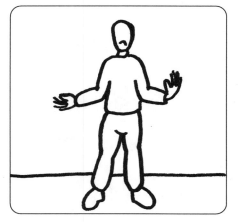

Incorrect

➤ Rotator Cuff Rotation:

Standing with your feet shoulder width apart and your arms out to the side raised to shoulder height, bend your elbows, with hands pointing toward the ceiling. Slowly rotate your hands and forearms forward, palms facing toward the floor. Rotate them back up until pointing toward the ceiling. If you can't coordinate two arms at the same time, do each arm separately. Build to 10 repetitions.

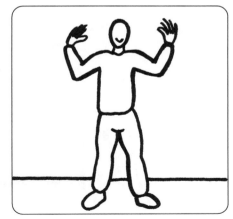

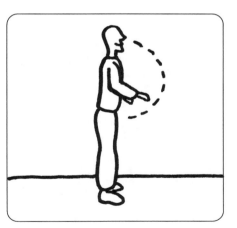

 Front View

 Side View

➤ Fly Like a Bird:

Standing with your feet shoulder width apart, and your hands down at your side, palms facing the sides of your legs, raise your arms upward and outward to shoulder height. Return your arms to the hanging position. If you can't coordinate both arms to move at the same time, do each arm separately. Build up to 10 repetitions.

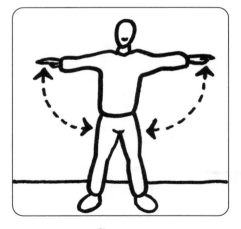

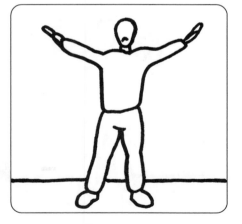

Correct   Incorrect

➤ Forward Arm Lifts:

Standing with feet shoulder width apart, your knees slightly bent and hands down at your sides, with your palms facing the back of your body, raise your arms upward and forward to shoulder height. Return your arms to the hanging position. If you can't coordinate both of your arms to raise at the same time, do each arm separately. Build up to 10 repetitions.

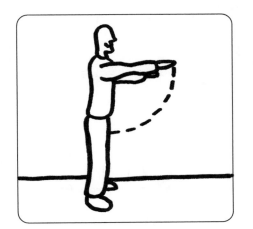

Side View

➤ Biceps Curls, Palms Down:

Either standing or sitting, with your arms hanging down at your side **and your elbows held tightly against your body**, and your palms facing backward, bring your hands upward toward your shoulders, and return them to the hanging position. (Back of hand will face shoulder when lifted up). Attempt to touch your shoulders with the backs of your hands. Do each arm separately if necessary. Build to 10 repetitions.

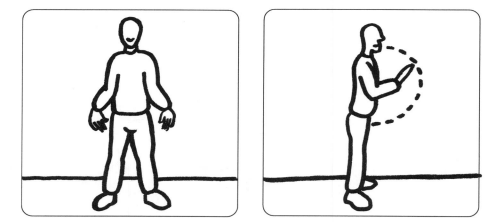

Front View   Side View

➤ Biceps Curls, Palms Up:

Repeat above exercise with your palms facing forward. (Palms will face shoulder when lifted up). Try to touch shoulders with the palms of your hands. Build to 10 repetitions.

➤ Arms, Opening a Door Knob:

Standing with shoulder width apart or sitting, and with arms held straight and stiff down at your side, your palms facing the side of your legs with thumbs toward the front of your body. Rotate your hands and arms as far inward as they will go. Your palms will face away from the side of your body with thumbs pointing toward the back. Then rotate your hands and arms around the other way as far as they will go. Again, your palms will face away from the side of your body. The motion will be as if you are opening a door knob. One inward rotation and one return rotation = one repetition. Build to 10 repetitions. Do each arm separately if necessary.

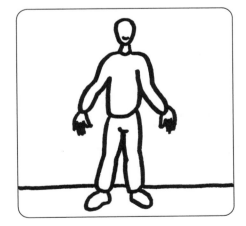

Inward Rotations

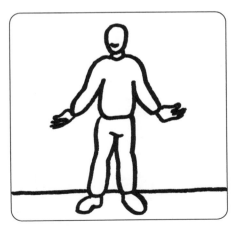

Outward Rotations

➤ Hand, Inside and Outside Circles:

Either sitting or standing, with elbows at your side and your arms bent to a 90 degree angle, rotate your hands in circles rotating inward. **Keep your forearm stable.** Make as big a circle as you can. Do each wrist separately if moving them simultaneously is difficult. Build to 10 circles. Repeat, rotating your hands in outward circles. Build to 10 circles.

➤ Hand Lifts:

Sitting with elbows at side and forearm supported either on table top, chair arm, or standing with wrist held underneath with opposite hand, and your **palm facing down**, slowly pull fingers of right hand upward as far as you can. Spread and hyperextend your fingers. Return to flat position. If you can't raise your hand without assistance, use your free hand to gently pull your fingers and hand upward or have some assistance in applying gentle pressure to your hand. Build to 10 repetitions. Repeat with the left hand.

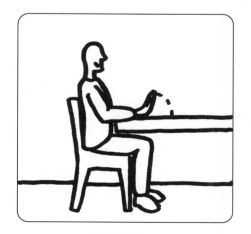

Side View

➤ Hands, Squeeze and Open:

Sitting or standing, squeeze your hand into a fist and open it flat, **with your fingers spread. Make your hand perfectly flat between fists.** Do each hand separately if doing the two simultaneously is difficult. Build to 10 repetitions.

➤ Finger Pinching:

Sitting or standing, pinch your first finger and thumb of your right hand together, then **open to a flat hand with fingers spread apart.** Build to 10 pinches. Repeat pinching with middle, ring and little fingers in succession. Repeat with your left hand fingers and thumb.

➤ Finger Drumming:

Sitting or standing with forearms on a table or counter top, drum your fingers in cadence, starting with your little finger and moving sequentially to your thumb. Do each hand separately if necessary to coordinate. Build to 10 repetitions.

➤ Finger Spreads:

Sitting or standing with forearms supported on table or counter top, alternately separate your fingers (spread them out) and return to normal position. Do each hand separately, if necessary. Build to 10 repetitions.

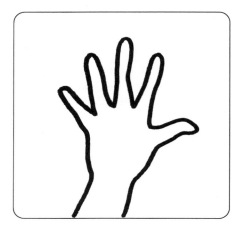 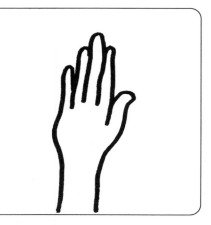

Fingers Spread   Normal

➤ Shoulder Stretches, Forward

Sitting or standing, with left arm at shoulder height, elbow slightly bent, use your right arm holding under your left elbow to pull your left arm across your body close to your chest to stretch your left shoulder. Hold for a count of 5. Let arms hang straight down. Raise your right arm to shoulder height, with your left arm holding your right arm under the elbow, pull your right arm across your body close to your chest to stretch your right shoulder. Hold for a count of 5. Relax your arms. One repetition only.

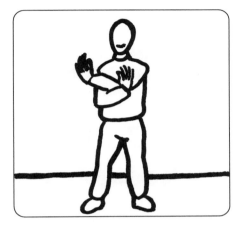

Right Stretch

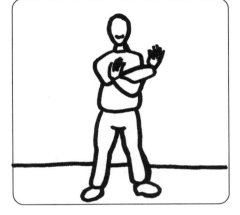

Left Stretch

➤ Shoulder Stretches, Backward:

Standing, or sitting on a stool or bench, clasp your hands together behind your back with arms straight. Pull your shoulder blades together in back, while stretching downward with your clasped hands. Let your chin fall to your chest and hold to a count of 5. Relax. One repetition only.

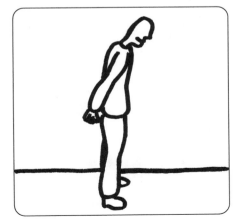

Side View

➤ Leg Circles, Inside:

Standing at a counter top or holding sturdy chair back, holding your right leg slightly outward and straight, draw a circle on the floor with your right foot, rotating counterclockwise or inside rotation. Make as large a circle as is comfortable. Build up to 10 rotations. Repeat this exercise with your left leg, rotating your leg clockwise, to do inside rotations.

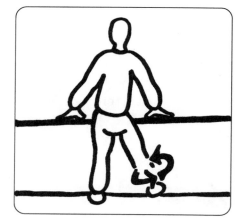

Right Leg   Left Leg

➤ Leg Circles, Outside:

Repeat above exercise doing outside rotations or circles. Again, do each leg separately, and build up to 10 rotations.

➤ Leg Slides, Outside:

Standing at counter top or holding sturdy chair back, shift
your weight to your left leg. Keeping your right leg straight,
slide your foot to the right as far as is comfortable and slide
it back. Build up to 10 slides. Repeat with the left leg.

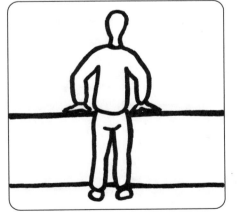

Beginning

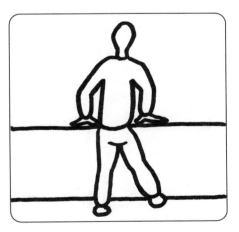

Progressing

➤ Leg Slides, Crossover:

Do not do this exercise if you have had hip replacement surgery without getting permission from your orthopedic surgeon. Standing at a counter top or holding onto sturdy chair back, shift your weight to your left leg. Slide your right foot in front of your left foot across your body and slide it back. Build to 10 slides. Repeat with the left leg crossing in front of your right foot.

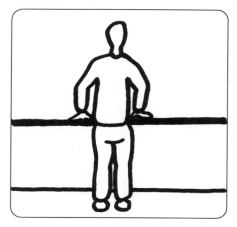
Beginning

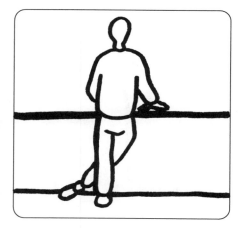
Progressing

➤ Foot Up and Down:

Preferably while standing at a counter top or holding onto sturdy chair back, shift your weight to your left leg. Place your right foot slightly forward from your left. Pull your right toes upward, flexing your ankle. Keep your heel on the ground. Raise your foot up and down. **Keep your posture erect.** Build up to 10 raises. Shift your weight to the right foot, place your left foot slightly forward, and do the foot up and down motion with your left foot.

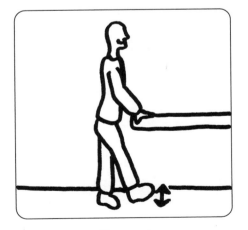

Correct

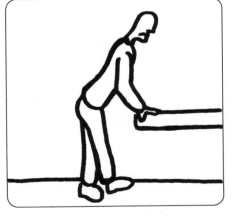

Incorrect

➤ Foot, Inside Circles:

Standing at a counter top or holding onto sturdy chair back, shift your weight to your left foot. Placing your right foot slightly ahead of your left, keeping the heel of your right foot firmly on the ground, rotate your foot up, toward the inside, down, toward the outside and back up, making inside circles. Build up to 10 rotations. Shift your weight to the right leg, place your left foot slightly in front of your right, and do the exercise with your left foot.

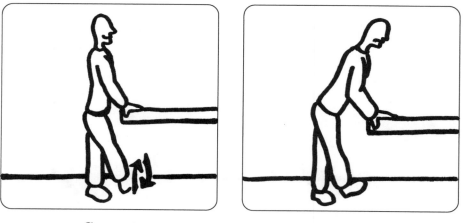

Correct   Incorrect

➤ Foot, Outside Circles:

Repeat the above exercise, but this time rotate your foot toward the outside by lifting up, moving toward the outside, down, toward the inside, and up. Build up to 10 rotations. Shift your weight to the right foot and do the exercise with your left foot.

Stretching and Cool-Down Exercises

➤ Front Leg (quadriceps) Stretch:

Standing in front of a counter or sturdy chair back step backward as far as is comfortable with your right foot, bending your left knee, and keeping your right leg straight. **Do not let your left knee go beyond your toes. Keep upright posture.** Place your right heel on the floor and count to 5. Move right foot back to normal standing position. Repeat exercise stepping back with your left foot. Do one repetition only.

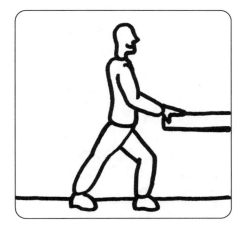

Correct

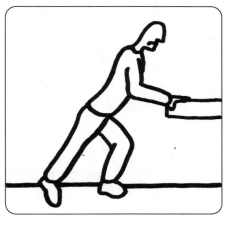

Incorrect

➤ Back Leg (hamstring) Stretch:

Standing in front of a counter or sturdy chair back, step back with your right foot, keeping your right heel on the ground. Bend your right knee, and bend forward from the buttocks, reaching your buttocks backward. Raise your left toes off the ground, keeping your heel on the ground, and your left leg straight. Hold to a count of 5. Return your right foot to a normal standing position. Repeat the exercise, stepping back with your left foot. Do one repetition only.

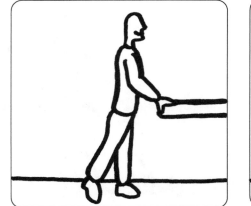

Position 1

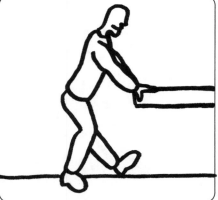

Position 2

➤ Sideways Leg Stretches:

Standing in front of a counter or sturdy chair back, spread your legs apart as far as is comfortable. Keeping your left foot facing forward, turn your right foot and torso to the right until you are at a 90 degree angle from the counter or chair back. **Keep your trunk erect—do not bend forward.** Stretch your right knee forward until it is over your toes. **Do not stretch your knees beyond your toes.** Hold to a count of 5. Turn your right foot back until it is facing forward. Repeat the exercise keeping your right foot forward and rotating your left foot and torso to the left until your left foot is 90 degrees from the counter.

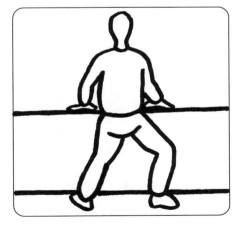 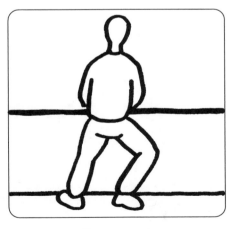

Correct   Incorrect

➤ Monkey Hang:

Standing in front of a sofa or large upholstered chair and with **someone else standing next to you,** with your feet shoulder width apart and your **knees slightly bent,** lean forward, reaching toward the floor with your arms. Let the top of your head come down, and hang relaxed, stretching the backs of your legs and your back. Do not attempt to stretch to reach the floor. Just hang relaxed. Hold to a count of 5.

Note:

If you have severe osteoporosis do not do this exercise!

If you have hypertension (high blood pressure) do not let your head go below waist level. If you need to, let your hands rest lightly on the seat of the sofa to maintain balance.

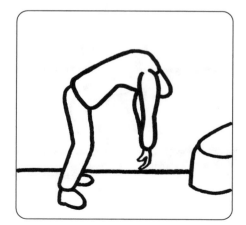

Correct

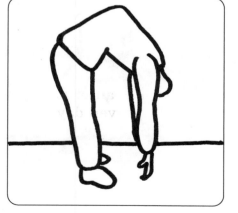

Incorrect

APPENDIX E3:
AEROBIC EXERCISES

NOTE: **DO NOT UNDERTAKE ANY TYPE OF EXERCISE ACTIVITY WITHOUT APPROVAL OF YOUR PHYSICIAN!**

Frequency: Preferably daily, but at least 3 times per week

When: After doing warm up exercises from Appendix E2 pages 175-181

Aerobic Exercise Information:

Some form of aerobic exercise should be performed minimally three times per week. These activities should be spaced throughout the week, e.g., Monday, Wednesday and Friday. However, daily aerobic exercise will reduce stress and anxiety and give the person with dementing illness a sense of well-being, as well as improving cardiovascular fitness (heart and lung fitness) and physical endurance. It may be a welcome break to exercise six rather than seven days a week. Cardiovascular fitness will not be lost with one day of rest between exercise sessions.

Warm up, range of motion, and stretching exercises should always be completed before starting any type of aerobic activity.

Generally, gentle, repetitive activities which increase the heart rate for 20 minutes are safe for most older persons. There is increasing evidence that shorter periods of aerobic activity two or three times a day will be beneficial, as well. **If there is any evidence of pain, increased shortness of breath, or excessive sweating, exercise should be stopped immediately.**

If the person is not accustomed to aerobic activity, the length of exercise time must be increased gradually. Usually, starting with 5 minutes per day for the first week, then increasing the time by 5 minutes on a weekly basis up to a total of 20 to 30 minutes daily, will be gradual enough for the older adult to adapt without creating any undue physical stress.

Several different activities may be aerobic in nature for the aging adult. Walking, dancing, riding a stationary exercise bicycle (without increased tension), and no-impact gentle aerobic exercise routines will all be effective. Generally, ski machines and stair climbers require too much exertion for the older adult. But if the person is accustomed to vigorous exercise, there is no reason to stop because of dementing illness. It is important to find an activity or combination of activities that are enjoyed by the person with dementia.

Aerobic exercise works best if there is consistent, repetitive motion. Therefore, if utilizing an exercise bike or dancing, there should be no fast spurts of activity followed by rests. Rather, a slow, consistent pace should be maintained throughout the 20-30 minute period.

Usually walking, even slow walking, is aerobic for the aging adult. Calculation of the heart rate necessary to maintain an aerobic state is different for the aging adult. As age increases, the heart rate necessary to perform aerobically decreases. **Generally, a 10 second pulse rate between 15 and 20 will be more than adequate to sustain aerobic functioning in any adult between the ages of 70 and 90**. Going beyond this range is not safe for the older adult. Check the pulse rate of the person with dementing illness every 5 minutes for a 10 second period. If the heart rate increases above the suggested range, slow the pace until it goes back in range.

If you are having difficulty calculating a pulse rate, use two simple indicators to determine if you are overworking. The first is a simple talk test. If you are able to say a phrase without gasping for breath, you are not overworking. The second is simply noting the way you feel. If you feel you are overexerting and short of breath, slow your pace and your activity until you are more comfortable.

Once aerobic exercise is completed, do not stop suddenly. Just walk slowly for a minute or so to allow the body to cool down. Then perform the stretching and cool-down exercises found in Appendix E2 starting on page 201.

APPENDIX E4:
TONING EXERCISES

NOTE: DO NOT UNDERTAKE ANY TYPE OF EXERCISE ACTIVITY WITHOUT APPROVAL OF YOUR PHYSICIAN!

Frequency: 3 times per week with a day of rest between (e.g., Monday, Wednesday, Friday)

When: After doing warm up and balance exercises pages 175-181.

Toning exercises are important to strengthen muscles which get used less and less as we age. Weak muscles contribute to balance problems, postural problems, elimination problems, and potential for falls.

To reduce the potential for injury, **do not do these exercises without first doing the warm up and balance exercises, pages 175-181.** Ideally, these exercises should be done after completing the entire range of motion exercise section, pages

182-200. However, I realize this may be too long a sequence for some people.

Some of these exercises are done standing. Some are done sitting. When choosing something on which to sit, choose a small chair with no arms, such as a dining room chair, or a piano stool or bench, to allow for movement of the arms and stretching of the sides. **Be certain your feet can sit firmly and flatly on the floor** when sitting.

Some of these exercises require getting down on the floor. If you cannot get both down and up, do not do these exercises. After a few months of working with the entire exercise segment you may gain enough strength to get down to the floor to do these exercises. Please, **to prevent injury, do not attempt to do these exercises on a bed or couch.** Be certain you do these exercises on a carpet, or preferably, on an exercise mat on a carpet, to prevent injury.

If your muscles are not in good shape and you have not been a regular exerciser, work only on the exercises found in sections E2 and E3 until you can do these exercises with relative ease. This may take up to 2 months.

When starting this segment, do so without weights (for the exercises requiring them) and gradually work up to doing all repetitions before adding weights. Choose the type of weight that is most comfortable for you. Hand held weights are fine, or you may prefer stretchable wrist or ankle weights. Probably the most flexible are the wraparound weights to which you can add additional weight as you desire. When you begin adding weights, start with a smaller number of repetitions and gradually build up to the complete sequence once again. Start with $\frac{1}{2}$ pound or 1 pound weights until all repetitions can be completed. Then advance to 2 pound, 3 pound, or 5 pound weights, if you desire, again doing a smaller number of repetitions and building to the complete sequence. One pound weights may be all that are needed, especially for women. I would not recommend going above 3 pound weights for women, and 5 pound weights for the very strong man.

The important part of toning exercise is not to do the exercises quickly, but rather to do them very slowly in both directions. The up movements and the down movements are equally important.

➤ Biceps Curls—use weights

Either standing with feet shoulder width apart and knees slightly bent, or sitting on a chair without arms, keeping your elbows tightly against the sides of your body, and your palms facing upward, slowly move your forearms up toward your shoulder and down to your feet. **Keep your elbow slightly bent when arm is completely lowered**. Do not hyperextend your elbow joint. Move slowly and steadily in both directions. Build to 10 repetitions.

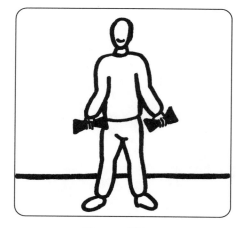

Front View

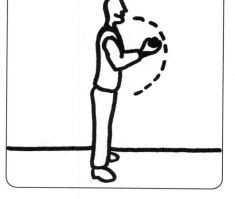

Side View

➤ Triceps—Little Lifts—use weights

Either standing with feet should width apart with knees
slightly bent, or sitting on a seat without arms or back, lean
forward slightly. With your arms down at your side and your
palms facing backwards and your arms held straight and
stiff, push or lift your arms backwards in little controlled
movements. Move slowly and deliberately. Weights can be on
each arm, or alternatively, use a piece of doweling or round
stick and hang a flexible weight over the stick. Build to 10
repetitions. Hold the last repetition to a count of 5.

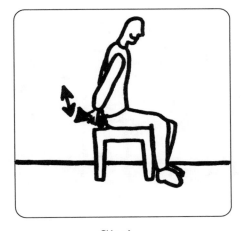

Sitting

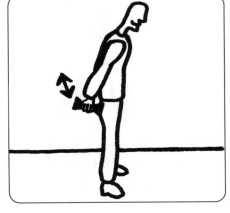

Standing

➤ Deltoids Side—use weights

Either standing with feet shoulder width apart and knees slightly bent, or sitting on seat without arms or back, let your arms hang down at your sides with palms facing the side of your legs. Slowly lift your arms up and down sideways, as if flying like a bird. Go slowly up and slowly down. **Do not go above shoulder height.** Build to 10 repetitions. Hold the last repetition to a count of 5 when your arms have reached shoulder height.

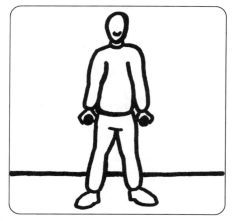

Position 1

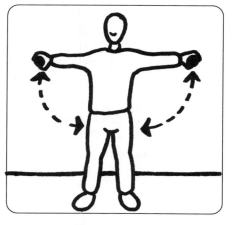

Position 2

➤ Deltoids Front—use weights

Either standing with your feet shoulder width apart and your knees slightly bent, or sitting on a seat without arms or a back, let your arms hang down at your side with palms facing backward. Slowly lift your straight arms up and forward to shoulder height and slowly down. Build to 10 repetitions. The last repetition hold to a count of 5 when arms are at shoulder height. Either use a weight on each arm or alternatively hold a round stick between your two hands with a weight hanging in the middle.

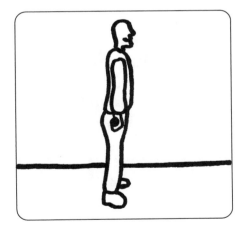

Position 1

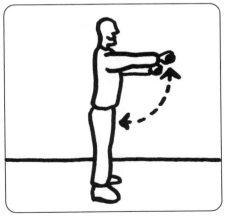

Position 2

➤ Upper Back—use weights

If you have balance problems, do this exercise sitting. Either
standing with your feet shoulder width apart and knees bent
or sitting on a seat without arms or back, lean as far forward
as is comfortable. With your elbows close to your side and
bent at a 90 degree angle, slowly move your elbows backward, pinching your shoulder blades together as you do so.
Move your elbows back to the starting position. Build up to
10 repetitions.

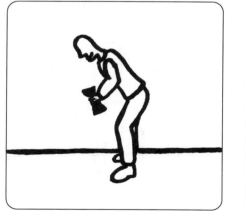

Position 1

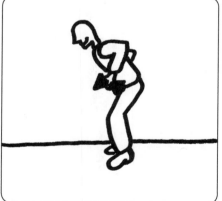

Position 2

➤ Chest Push and Pull—use weights

Either standing with feet shoulder width apart and knees slightly bent, or sitting on a seat with no arms or back, with your elbows close to your body, raise your forearms up so your hands are **at chest height**, palms facing forward. Slowly push your arms out and forward at chest height and slowly pull them back toward your chest, using your chest muscles and your upper back muscles and keeping your elbows tightly against your side. Build to 10 repetitions.

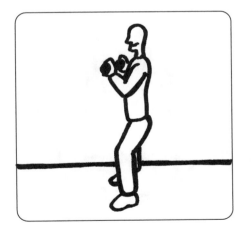 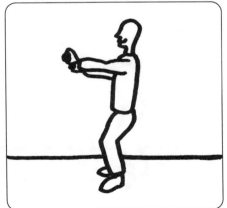

Position 1   Position 2

➤ Chest Squeezes—use weights

Either standing with your feet shoulder width apart and knees slightly bent, or sitting on a seat with no arms or back, raise your arms outward and forward until they are directly in front of you at **chest height**. Turn your hands so your palms are facing each other, toward the center. Act as if you are playing an accordian, slowly squeezing your straight arms in and out in little movements, contracting your arm muscles with each movement. Squeeze with your chest muscles as you are pulling your arms inward. Build to 10 squeezes.

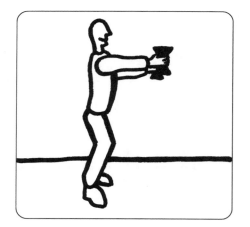

Side View

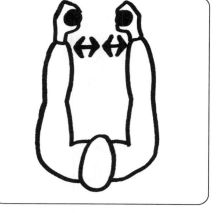

Overhead View

➤ Chest Stretch

Standing with feet shoulder width apart or sitting on stool with no back, clasp your hands behind your buttocks. Pull your shoulders backward and downward, pulling your shoulder blades together in back, to stretch your chest muscles. Hold to a count of 10.

➤ Big Hug

Give yourself a big hug. You deserve it!

Pull your shoulders forward and hold to a count of 10 to stretch your hard worked muscles.

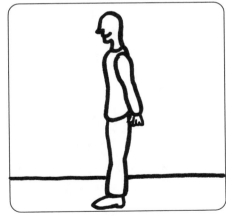

Chest Stretch

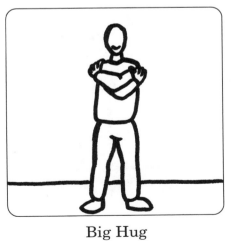

Big Hug

➤ Side Pulls—no weights

Standing with your feet shoulder width apart with knees slightly bent or sitting at the edge of a narrow seat without arms or back, slowly lean sideways to the right as far as you can reaching toward the floor with your right hand, and bringing your left hand up your left side. **Do not lean forward**, bend directly sideways. Then reverse the pull. Pulling your right hand up your right side and leaning to the left and reaching downward with your left hand. Right pull + left pull = one repetition. Build to 10 repetitions.

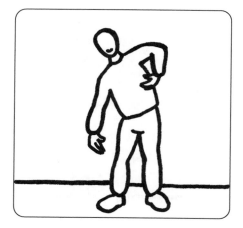
Right Side Pull

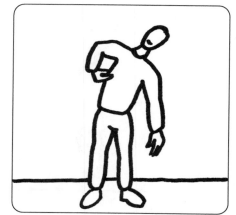
Left Side Pull

➤ Slight Knee Bends—no weights

Standing with your back against a wall with your feet shoulder width apart and your heels approximately 8-10 inches from the wall, and keeping your buttocks, small of your back, and shoulders against the wall, slide downward slightly, bending your knees. Do not let your knees extend beyond your toes. Push up to a standing position. Slowly go up and down. Build up to 10 repetitions. Hold the last bend to a count of 10.

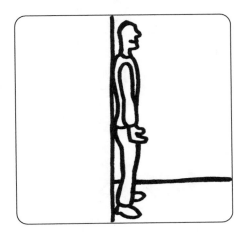

Standing

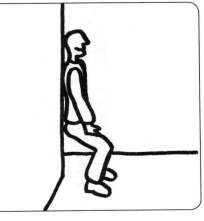

Squatting

➤ Buttocks Squeeze—no weights

Standing with your back against a wall with your feet shoulder width apart, your knees slightly bent and your heels approximately 4 inches from the wall, press the small of your back into the wall, squeezing your buttocks and back of your legs tightly together. Slowly press, squeeze and relax. Build to 10 repetitions. Hold the last press and squeeze to a count of 5.

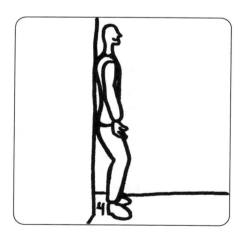

Relaxed Position

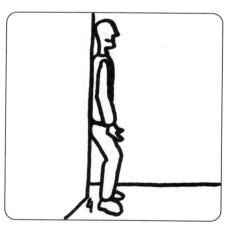

Pressed and Squeezed Position

➤ Side Leg Lifts—no weights

Standing facing a kitchen counter with feet shoulder width apart and knees slightly bent, slowly raise your right leg sideways to the right and slowly return it to the standing position. **Do not bend forward.** Build to 10 lifts. Hold to a count of 5 on your last lift.

Repeat sequence lifting the left leg.

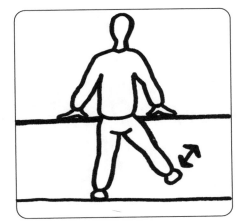
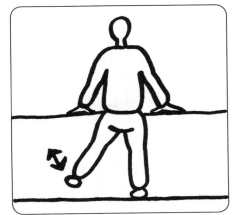

Right Side Lift   Left Side Lift

➤ Back Leg Lifts—no weights

Standing facing a kitchen counter with feet shoulder width apart and knees slightly bent and **remaining in an upright posture**, slowly lift the right leg backwards and slowly return it to the standing position. Build to 10 lifts. Hold to a count of 5 on the last lift.

Repeat sequence lifting the left leg.

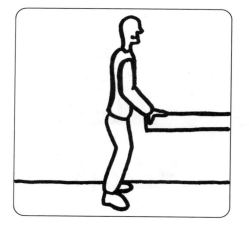
Position 1

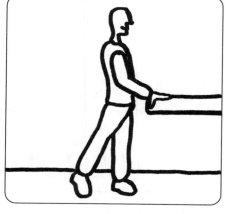
Position 2

➤ Heels and Toes—no weights

Standing facing a kitchen counter in case you need it for balance, with your feet shoulder width apart and your knees slightly bent and **your toes facing forward**, go up on your toes, **keeping your posture erect**. Do not lean forward. Keeping your posture erect (do not extend your buttocks outward) go down to standing position and rock back to standing on your heels (pull your toes up). Build to 5 repetitions.

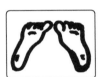

Repeat sequence with your toes turned outward.

Repeat sequence with your toes turned inward.

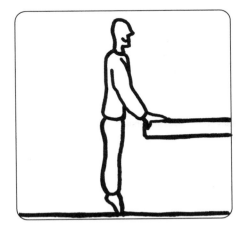
Toes

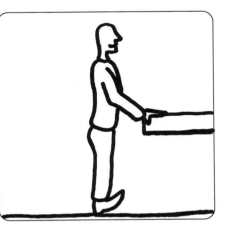
Heels

➤ Quadriceps Strengthening—no weights

Sitting on a seat with no arms, your feet firmly on the ground, and forward enough on the seat so the edge of seat is about at mid-thigh, hold your right leg up parallel to the floor with your toes pointed toward the ceiling to a count of 10. You may do foot circles for something to do if you wish. Repeat with the left leg.

Repeat exercise with first the right leg, then the left leg, with foot rotated outward and leg slightly bent.

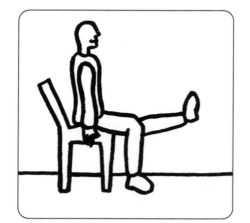

Side View

➤ Quadriceps with Bent Leg

Sitting on a chair seat with no arms, positioned toward the front of the seat with edge of seat hitting at mid-thigh and feet firmly on the ground, raise your right leg, with bent knee and foot directly in front of knee. Hold to a count of 10. Do only one repetition.

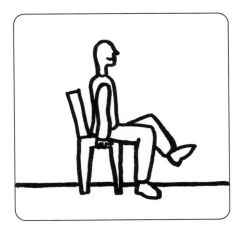

Side View

Repeat with the left leg.

➤ Back Stretch

Scoot back on your seat, and sitting with your feet firmly on the ground and feet shoulder width apart, hang forward, with your hands reaching toward the floor. Just hang there to a count of 10 and relax, stretching your back. One repetition only.

If you cannot get down on or up from the floor, you have completed the toning segment. Do the stretching exercises on pages 201-204. Stretching will keep your muscles from becoming sore.

If you can do some work on the floor, complete the following segment before doing the stretching exercises on pages 201-204. Be certain you are on a soft carpet or on an exercise mat placed on the carpet.

➤ Upper Abdomen

Lying on your back with your knees bent and your feet shoulder width apart and flat on the floor, place your hands behind and underneath your head if you can. If you can't put your hands behind your head, just leave them resting on your chest. Slowly raise your chin, nose, and shoulders straight upward toward the ceiling. You will feel the pull of the muscles in your upper abdomen. Just do **slight (2-4 inches)** movements up and down. Build to 10 repetitions.

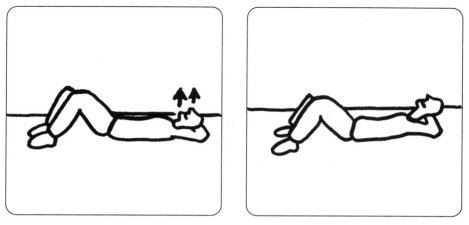

Position 1   Position 2

➤ Side Abdomen

Lying on your back on the floor with your knees bent and your feet together and firmly on the ground and your arms positioned as they were in the previous exercise, rotate your knees to the right and leave them there. Lift your chin, nose, and shoulders slowly slightly off the floor and slowly return to the resting position. You should feel your side abdominal muscles pulling. Keeping your knees to the right, build to 10 repetitions.

Turn your knees to the left and repeat the sequence.

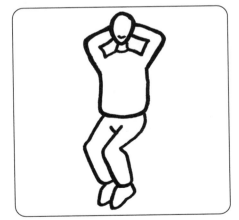

Top View

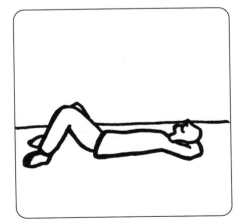

Side View

➤ Lower Abdomen

Lying on your back on the floor with your knees bent, place your hands, palms down on the floor, underneath your buttocks to provide protection for your back. Lift your knees and feet upward so your feet are slightly higher than your knees. Make **little (about 6 inches)** movements pulling your legs toward your head, pulling with your lower abdominal muscles. Do not place your feet back on the floor each time. Do the movements slowly. Build to 10 repetitions.

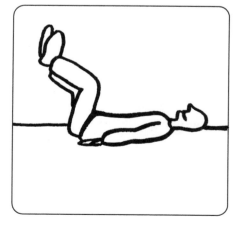

Position 1

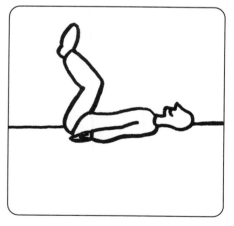

Position 2

> Back Bridge

Lying on your back with your knees bent, your heels as close to your buttocks as you can get them, your feet shoulder width apart, and your knees braced together, slowly lift your buttocks completely off the floor, placing your weight on your feet and your shoulders. Make a bridge with your body. Hold to a count of 5. Then, **slowly roll back down to the floor, vertebra by vertebra**. Build to 5 repetitions.

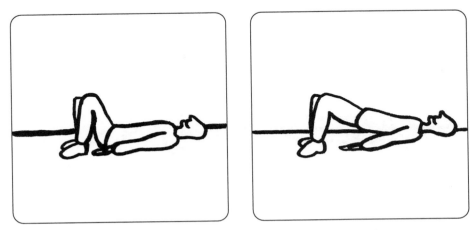

Position 1   Position 2

➤ Back Leg Stretches

Lying on your back on the floor with your knees bent and
your feet shoulder width apart, and your head and neck relaxed, raise your right leg toward the ceiling. Reach up and
hold behind your right thigh with your hands. Pull your leg
toward your head as far as is comfortable. Circle your feet if
you wish. Relax and enjoy the stretch to a count of 5. Place
your right foot back on the floor with knee bent.

Repeat the sequence raising your left leg.

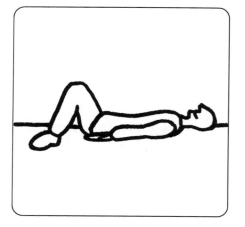

Position 1

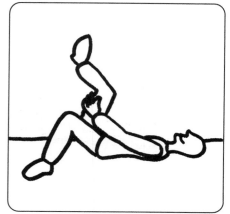

Position 2

➤ Back Stretch

Lying on the floor with your knees bent, slowly lift your right leg, reaching behind your leg with your hands and pulling it toward your face. Hold to a count of 5 and slowly return it to the floor.

Repeat lifting your left leg.

Repeat lifting both legs at once.

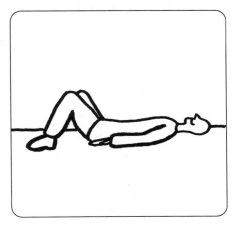

Starting Position

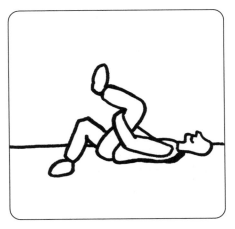

One Leg

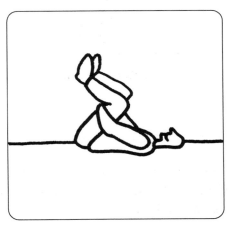

Both Legs

➤ Abdominal Stretches

Lying on the floor with your knees bent and your hands out
to your side, slowly roll your knees to the right while rolling
your head to the left. **Keep your shoulders firmly on the
floor.** Feel the stretch in your abdomen and back. Hold to a
count of 5. Slowly roll back onto your back. Then roll your
knees to the left while rolling your head to the right. Hold to
a count of 5 and slowly roll back onto your back.

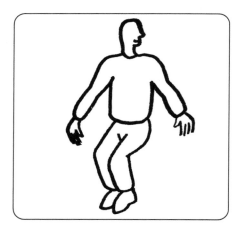   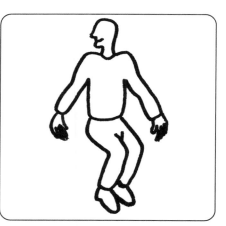

Knees to Right   Knees to Left

You are now finished with your toning exercises. Congratula-
tions! Please do the remainder of the stretching exercises on
pages 201-204.

ABOUT THE AUTHOR

Barbara Bridges was born and raised in the Seattle area of the Pacific Northwest. After receiving her nursing degree from the University of Washington, she served several years in the U.S. Navy Nurse Corps. Her clinical experiences have been in thoracic and cardiac surgery, coronary care units, and intensive care units. She has been a nursing administrator at major teaching hospitals in Southern California. Her graduate degrees are from California State University at Los Angeles and the University of Washington in Seattle.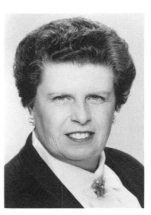

She spent fourteen years caring for her aging parents, both of whom had dementing illness. Barbara decided to author this book both not only to share her experiences with others, but also to fill what she feels is a void in information currently available to caregivers.

Barbara owns her own business, BJB Geriatric/Educational Services, providing in home consultation, family member caregiver training, and institutional caregiver training in the therapeutic management of persons with dementing illness. She presents at conferences and workshops nation-wide.

ORDERING INFORMATION

Comments Solicited:

I welcome your comments regarding this publication. Any suggestions for areas that need clarification or elaboration or suggestions for additions to content would be greatly appreciated. Phone calls or letters are welcome.

To Send Comments Write to:

Barbara J. Bridges
BJB Publishing
16212 Bothell Way S.E., Suite F171
Mill Creek, Washington 98012-1219

Phone: (800) 799-3414

Fax: (425) 338-0456

E-Mail: bjbservices@prodigy.net

To Place an Order:

Please refer to ordering information on the next page, or check your local book store or Alzheimer's Association office for immediate availability.

Therapeutic Caregiving Order Form

Multiple book orders: Call (800) 799-3414 for price information

Price:
Per book: $18.00
S&H: $ 3.50 book rate delivery
Priority: $ 1.00 additional for priority mail

To order:
Call: (800) 799-3414 with credit card information
Visa, Mastercard, or American Express only
E-Mail: bjbservices@prodigy.net or
Fax: (425) 338-0456 or
Web: http://pages.prodigy.com/bjbservices
Mail: Completed form with check, money order, or credit card information to:

BJB Publishing
16212 Bothell Way S.E., Suite F171
Mill Creek, Washington 98012-1219

Card Number: _ _ _ _ _ _ _ _ _ _ _ _ _ _ _ _

Expiration Date: _____/_____

Phone Number: (_____) _____

Name on Card: _____

Please print your complete mailing address below:

Name: _____

Organization: _____

Address: _____

City, State, Zip: _____

Phone: (_____) _____

Thank you for your order. Please allow 4 weeks for delivery.
Complete money back guarantee within 30 days of purchase.